CUBAN HEALTH CARE

CUBAN
HEALTH CARE

THE ONGOING REVOLUTION | DON FITZ

MONTHLY REVIEW PRESS

New York

Library of Congress Cataloging-in-Publication Data
available from the publisher

ISBN paper: 978-158367-860-2
ISBN cloth: 978-1-58367-861-9

On the cover: (top) Ward at Palacio de la Maternidad (Maternity Home), Cienfuegos, Cuba; (bottom) Cuban-trained medical student, Carlos Aldazabal, examines Peruvian girl, Lima, Peru. Photos by Don Fitz.

Typeset in Minion Pro and Gin

MONTHLY REVIEW PRESS, NEW YORK
monthlyreview.org

5 4 3 2 1

CONTENTS

CUBA SHOWS THAT CHANGE IS CONSTANT

When I first read Karl Marx as a teenager I questioned what socialism would look like and wondered why he did not spell it out as did
so many utopians of his time. I knew socialists who explained that
Marx avoided doing so because the process of struggle would lead to
new social formations, which would then become the building blocks
of post-capitalist societies. In the words of Ian Angus, "Fighting to
limit the danger caused by capitalism today will help lay the basis
for socialism tomorrow."[1] However, hearing such explanations in
my late teens still left me dubious. I wondered if "dialectical mate-
rialism" were nothing more than a way for socialists to camouflage
their lack of clarity about the type of social organization to come. As
I read more about the Paris Commune and especially the soviets of
the Russian Revolution, I was able to grasp why no one can seriously
make blueprints for a revolution's outcome. Instead, one can only
sketch the broad outlines of a new society, because those building it
will complete the details.

My role changed as years went by and I began explaining to others
that, as a revolution copes with unforeseen problems, it must develop
new solutions and incorporate them into social relationships in
ways that could barely be imagined in the old society. One day my

daughter Rebecca phoned after visiting Cuba to tell me that she'd
heard of a medical school there that attracted students from all over
the world. Soon she decided that she wanted to attend, and I gave
her my encouragement. I became increasingly fascinated with Cuba's
medical system, which I discovered was at least as remarkable as the
country's agricultural innovations that I had heard so much about.
Delving into Cuban medicine led me to realize that it beautifully
demonstrates how fulfilling the goals of the 1959 revolution brought
forth novel institutions which, interacting with forces both inside and
outside Cuban society, led to innovations that could not have been
conceived prior to the revolution.

Cuba had three medical revolutions before 1959: the first (from
1790 to 1830) focused on smallpox vaccination and sanitation; the
second (from 1898 to 1922) centered on immunization against yellow
fever; the third (from 1925 to 1945) brought a heightened awareness
of the relationship between poverty and disease. The goals of the third
revolution were fulfilled only after 1959, as the new government realized that providing preventive medicine to rural as well as urban areas
required reorganizing the delivery of care.[2] Chapter 1 of this book,
"The Three Thousand Who Stayed," describes the tasks of those Cuban
doctors who did not emigrate to Florida or elsewhere but remained to
expand medical services, build a unified health system, and redesign
medical education as they learned the role of mass mobilization in
effecting changes.

At the time of the Cuban revolution, much of the world was well
aware that the "actually existing socialism" in the USSR was no longer
an inspirational force. As Michael Lebowitz writes, "Real socialism
had not produced the new human beings who could build a better
world."[3] The physician Ernesto "Che" Guevara was key in inspiring the
Cuban revolution to recognize that socialism required the creation
of the "new man," for whom ethical motives prevailed over material
ones. In the early 1960s, revolutionary doctors challenged the ideology and practice of the former neocolonial regime by extending
medical care beyond the western urban center of Havana, which was
predominantly white, to areas that were mainly rural, more black, and

closer to Haiti in the eastern part of the island. They also planted the
seeds of internationalism with the first medical mission to Algeria
in 1963. The initial stage of medical transformation in Cuba, then,
involved the expansion not just of care but of medical consciousness,
which became a material force shaping the country's health system.

Overcoming the former system's racist and classist discrimination required confronting the contradiction that egalitarian health
care could not be attained within systems that were inherited from
capitalism. The way that Cuba addressed the contradiction between
the revolution's anti-capitalist goals and the residual capitalist structures in the island is the topic of chapter 2, "The Birth of the Cuban
Polyclinic." Numerous clinics, or *policlínicos*, as they are called in Latin
America, existed in Cuba alongside other caregiving structures, each
providing distinct services and using its own record-keeping system.
Beginning in 1964, *policlínicos integrales,* or comprehensive polyclinics, all with similar structures, were integrated into a nationwide
medical system. Each serving a defined geographic area, the *policlínicos integrales* provided distinct points of entry into the medical
system and vastly reduced the previous chaos of multiple independent providers. Although the policlinics had borrowed many ideas
from Soviet bloc countries, they were more decentralized. In great
measure, this was due to their independence from hospitals. Average
Cubans came to hold the policlinics in high esteem because of their
role in coordinating mass health campaigns.

Though the *policlínicos integrales* addressed the most serious internal problems of Cuban medicine, the sharp contrast between the mass
care provided on the island and the dire situation of the rest of the
world's poor countries loomed large. The Cuban military carried out
secret missions that were accompanied by doctors to support African
uprisings in the early 1960s. The role of Cuban medical staff during
its early forays into Africa is the subject of this book's third chapter,
"Cuba's First Military Doctors." Those doctors, who were often unaccustomed to dangerous field conditions, now had to perform under
the stress of enemy fire. They gained considerable knowledge about
treating diseases they had not previously known. Racial differences

that had tormented Cuba before the revolution saw a strange twist of roles between doctors and soldiers aboard ships to Africa. By the end of the 1960s, Cuban doctors had had four very different African experiences: in Algeria, they had treated only civilians; in Zaire,[4] the doctors had been disappointed by rebels who showed little enthusiasm for victory; in the Congo, they heard government proclamations which proved to be empty rhetoric; in Guinea Bissau, however, they had felt the satisfaction of working with a successful insurrectional movement with a strong commander and dedicated troops.

Inside Cuba, the innovations of the 1970s and 1980s relied heavily on what doctors had learned in the 1960s. Oddly enough, placing polyclinics in communities gave rise to an understanding of their limitations in providing genuine community health care. Chapter 4, "From *Policlínicos Comunitarios* to Family Doctors," describes how the internal inconsistencies of *policlínicos integrales* led to their complete redesign and their reemergence as *policlínicos comunitarios*. It also describes how contradictions within the latter resulted in the appearance of the Family Doctor/Nurse program. Though the *policlínicos integrales* had carried out a herculean task in bringing together disconnected services into a unified health care system, they were still insufficiently connected to the communities they were intended to serve. The shift to *policlínicos comunitarios* preserved the concept of the clinic being linked to a defined geographic area but added a critical element: in addition to people going to clinics, health professionals would now visit patients in their homes.

Polyclinics were reorganized so that specialists working together in teams would make home visits. As this system went into effect, practitioners discovered that despite its improvements, specialist teams of doctors and nurses were covering an area so large that they did not know patients well enough to anticipate impending problems. Then the revolutionary idea arose of creating doctor-and-nurse teams who would specialize in community medicine. These teams would live and work in areas small enough for them to walk to patient homes and monitor a variety of health-related problems simultaneously. The practice of doctor-and-nurse teams becoming a part of the community began in 1984. A novel residency training program played an important role in helping medical professionals combine coping with the most frequent daily problems and recognizing which symptoms required referral to a polyclinic or hospital.

As Cuba transformed its health system, the gap increased between the level of care of its citizens and the languishing medical situation of the newly independent African countries. Chapter 5, "Cuban Doctors in Angola," details campaigns in southern Africa in the 1970s and 1980s where doctors applied the knowledge gained during the medical missions of the 1960s to an enormously higher level of armed struggle. As Angola's independence from Portugal approached in 1974, three factions emerged: the Popular Movement for the Liberation of Angola (MPLA), which represented the country's only hope for autonomy, and two groups closely aligned with imperial powers. The medical situation was dire, since most doctors had fled Angola, with only fourteen remaining. After initially hesitating, Cuba answered Angola's call for military and medical aid. Then, following a major intervention by South Africa, Cuba rushed its soldiers and doctors to the Angolan front. As in the campaigns of the 1960s, Cuban doctors learned how to treat battle wounds and tropical diseases they had not seen at home. Now, however, their efforts were open rather than secret and the number returning home with these experiences would be much larger.

Though it appeared that the fighting might end by 1976, South Africa continued to send troops and pro-Western Angolans increased their attacks. There was, however, a lull, and Cuban doctors focused on helping civilians, treating injured combatants, and protecting themselves. During this time, tens of thousands of Cuban medical staff, teachers, and construction workers went to Angola and to dozens of other African countries, and to Asia, Latin America, and the Caribbean. In Angola, the lines were drawn between the MPLA, with Cuban and Soviet support, versus South Africa with its Angolan allies and U.S. support. The fighting reached a peak during the period 1985–88, with Fidel Castro conceiving military maneuvers that cleverly outwitted the supporters of apartheid. When Cuba's military left

Angola in June 1991, its aid workers, including doctors, were forced to leave too, because otherwise they would have been brutally attacked by pro-Western Angolans.

More than a third of a million Cubans returned at the end of the Angolan wars, and they were jolted by what confronted them. One was the global HIV/AIDS epidemic to which Cuba was particularly vulnerable. Could the island's medical system cope with it? Then, just when the country had modified its quarantine policy and established novel treatment approaches, another huge trial came with the December 1991 collapse of the Soviet Union. Previous medical challenges had been ones over which Cuba had a large degree of control because they either originated internally or were external events they chose to participate in. Chapter 6, "A Time of the Unexpected," focuses on how a health system developed during three decades of revolution confronted powers outside Cuba threatening to shatter its foundations.

With the fall of the Eastern bloc, the island lost its subsidies from the USSR, a large majority of its imports including oil, and most of its market for exports. This "Special Period in the Time of Peace," as it was called, affected people's health directly. At the same time, it hindered the state's ability to provide medical care as well as educate future professionals. Would Cuba be able to survive decreasing food supplies and shortcomings in daily hygiene and emergency care? As the AIDS crisis intensified globally, especially in southern Africa and the Caribbean, Cuban care delivery confronted its own homophobia, once again confirming that consciousness can become a material force. Rather than the positive form of consciousness of its own power being a material force in the liberation of the working class, consciousness in the form of prejudice proved to be a negative force by interfering with the quality of medical care for those with HIV/AIDS.

The tightening of the U.S. embargo caused Cubans to profoundly alter their daily lives, while the government, with great trepidation, began its own version of Lenin's New Economic Policy (NEP). That is, Cuba decided to allow tightly supervised mini-capitalism within a context of highly expanded tourism. Whereas some Bolsheviks had used the slogan "Get Rich!" during the NEP, the Cuban policies during the Special Period were more in line with a slogan like "Survive!" Health care services became a priority for revenue from other economic spheres. This, along with the egalitarian structure of Cuba's medical system, allowed the country not only to recover during the Special Period but even to improve medical indicators by the turn of the millennium. Along with direct care, medical institutions and research expanded.

At the same time, Cuba resumed its international aid programs, though in a variation that prioritized medical aid. In 1998, Hurricane Mitch slammed Central America, prompting a response from Cuba. That event set the stage for the biggest transformation thus far in the island's approach to global aid. After offering one thousand medical scholarships to students from the countries most ravaged by Mitch, Fidel and his medical advisers decided that Cuba should bring students from across the world to study medicine in a central location. This was the origin of the Latin American School of Medicine (ELAM, for its Spanish acronym) which chapters 7 and 8 explore. Chapter 7, "ELAM: The Latin American School of Medicine," tells how it had enrolled 21,018 medical students from over one hundred countries by 2010. The school's curriculum was carefully designed to help students serve their countries' most needy populations when they returned. ELAM drew on Cuba's vast experience working abroad and became a unifying force for future medical missions. Since so many people around the world rely on traditional and natural healers, the Cuban model of Comprehensive General Medicine (MGI, *Medicina General Integral*) teaches students to be listeners and healers as much as doctors. The ELAM curriculum differs according to whether students have sufficient pre-med background, whether they are from Cuba, Latin America, or a non-Latin culture, and whether they are fluent in Spanish. The chapter describes the culture of medical school in Havana, the base curriculum, and the interests of students coming from a variety of countries. Chapter 8, "Thirteen Faces of ELAM," looks more closely at international students attending the school.

Cuba is remaking medicine in a range of contexts: from Latin America and the Caribbean to Africa, Asia, and the Pacific Islands. Impossible to replicate in an exact fashion, the Cuban model must be adapted wherever it goes. Chapter 9, "Cuba: The New Global Medicine," features three in-depth accounts of ELAM students participating in community projects and international crisis relief. Following the 2007 earthquake in Peru, Cuban doctors faced multiple obstacles as they established *consultorios* and a *policlínico* in that country based on the Cuban model. In Haiti, relief efforts following the 2010 earthquake led to Haitian patients developing very different relationships with Cuban doctors than those they established with U.S. doctors. This chapter also looks at how a group of African and African-American medical students in Havana worked to blend Cuban medical approaches with traditional Ghanaian healing practices.

Chapter 10, "Challenges of the Twenty-First Century," looks at three important challenges Cuba has faced in recent times, then outlines some of the key lessons to be learned from the Cuban health model. The first part of the chapter, which relies on Steve Brouwer's *Revolutionary Doctors: How Venezeula and Cuba Are Changing the World's Conception of Health Care*, examines Venezuela's unique effort to reproduce the entire Cuban health system via the *Barrio Adentro* I through IV programs. It shows how a system, once developed, can be implemented elsewhere with structural changes introduced in the opposite order of their original appearance (though the Family Doctor/Nurse Program was the last step in the unfolding of the Cuban system, it was the first step in Venezuela). The second part of the chapter is based on my participation in Cuba's celebration of the 2012 March Against Homophobia. Any country with a homophobic history, including Cuba, must have mass participation in efforts to transform its culture if it is to remove barriers to effective health care. The third part of the chapter describes how Cuba worked to control dengue fever by actively involving the population. That approach reflects the country's history of mass mobilizations and is a model for poor countries needing a low-cost method for controlling mosquito-borne illnesses. The chapter also presents key lessons learned from the Cuban experience of health care reform.

Chapter 11, "Cuba's Medical Mission," takes stock of the country's health care endeavors during the second decade of this century. It describes Cuba's response to the Ebola virus panic of 2014; the medical services Cuba has provided to remote regions; the West's calculated underreporting and baseless critiques of Cuba's accomplishments; and the contrast between Cuban internationalism and the "disaster tourism" more characteristic of U.S. medical missions abroad. The chapter also contrasts corporate use of biotechnology in the service of agroindustry giants such as Bayer/Monsanto to Cuban biotechnology research that aims to improve medicine in underserved countries.

Chapter 12 concerns the current structure of medical care inside Cuba and contrasts it with the U.S. system, whose bloated nature goes far beyond the powers of insurance companies. It covers the fragmented nature of health care reimbursement that employs a small army of gatekeepers. It also examines undertreatment, overtreatment of real and non-real illnesses, sickness "looping," pharmaceutical "looping," over-diagnosing, pharmaceutical overpricing, intentional pharmaceutical waste and profiteering in what could be called the "sickness industry."

Though the U.S. system is often criticized by contrasting it to other rich countries, it should also be compared to the Cuban health care system, which is more sustainable and holistic. Chapter 12 also examines the non-financial aspects of corporate medicine, including unnecessary pain and avoidable deaths. Can the problems with U.S. health care be resolved by "Medicare-for-All," which follows the European model? Cuban medicine was born in the context of a complete reconceptualization of society. Its success shows that medicine must be a critical component in a bigger picture of overcoming multiple forms of oppression.

ACKNOWLEDGMENTS

Completing this book was not a solitary project. It was only possible due to the assistance of dozens of people. Before referring to them, I want to recognize the works that helped me form a broad view of the Cuban medical project. Ross Danielson's *Cuban Medicine* (1979) chronicles the various medical revolutions in Cuba, from the earliest known times through the development of polyclinics. Two works by Piero Gleijeses, *Conflicting Missions: Havana, Washington, and Africa, 1959–1976* (2002) and *Visions of Freedom: Havana, Washington, Pretoria, and the Struggle for Southern Africa, 1976–1991* (2013), thoroughly document Cuba's role in Africa. *Cuba, Revolución Social y Salud Pública: 1959–1984* (2008) by José R. Ruíz Hernández, often read by Cuban students, is the official history of the health system from the first days of the revolution through the development of family medicine.

Breaking the decades of silence that Cuba maintained on its medical missions in Africa, the 2005 publication of Hedelberto López Blanch's *Historias Secretas de Médicos Cubanos* collects oral histories of doctors' experiences in Algeria in 1963 through the 1975 battles in Angola. Linda M. Whiteford and Lawrence G. Branch's *Primary Health Care in Cuba: The Other Revolution* (2008) is one of the most readable short books that captures the essentials of Cuban health care. By contrast, Stan Cox's *Sick Planet: Corporate Food and Medicine* (2008) succinctly documents the effects of medicine as a business in the United States. Two books by John M. Kirk, *Cuban Medical Internationalism: Origins, Evolution and Goals* (2009), co-authored by Michael H. Erisman, and *Health Care without Borders: Understanding Cuban Medical Internationalism* (2015), constitute the definitive accounts of the work of Cuban doctors overseas. Anyone wishing to understand the story of two countries working in close partnership to change medicine to benefit the world's poor should read Steve Brouwer's *Revolutionary Doctors: How Venezuela and Cuba Are Changing the World's Conceptualization of Health Care* (2011).

My research depends heavily on interviews and oral histories, and I wish to thank the many people who shared their experiences with me. Dr. Ezno Dueñas Gómez and Dr. Felipe Cárdenas Gonzáles recounted the changes they witnessed while living through the revolution. Along with Dr. María Luísa Lima, they told me of the development of Cuba's first polyclinics. Dr. Justo Piñeiro described his experiences as a Cuban doctor in Tanzania from September 1966 to November 1967. I received firsthand accounts of the medical mission in Angola from Dr. Jorge Luís Martínez, Dr. Carlos Suárez Monteagudo, and Dr. Oscar Mena Hector.

I am also grateful to the ELAM students who granted me interviews, including those from the United States (Cassandra Cusack Curbelo, Omavi Bailey, and Ketia Brown), Mexico (Exa Gonzalez), Peru (Ivan Angulo Torres), Honduras (Anmnol Colindres), Brazil (Ivan Gomez de Assis and Walter Titz), Saint Lucia (Amanda Louis), Sierra Leone (Dennis Pratt), Kenya (Lorine Auma), Lesotho (Keitumetse Joyce Letsiela), São Tomé and Príncipe (Yell Eric), and Tuvalu (Jonalisa Livi Tapumanaia). Health care worker Teresa Frías, who has worked in Angola, Tanzania, Brazil, and Bolivia, guided me in my first visit to a Cuban polyclinic. At the first *consultorio* I visited in Havana, I interviewed Dr. Alejandro Fadragas Fernández and nurse Maité Perdomo. In the Peruvian city of Pisco, polyclinic director Leopoldo García Mejias explained to me how polyclinics function within that country's medical system. At *Consultorio* No. 2 in Pisco, I interviewed Dr. Johnny Carrillo Prada and Dr. María Concepción Paredes Huacoto.

To document the work of Cuba's doctors in Haiti after the 2010 earthquake, I spoke by phone with ELAM student Joanna Souers. Deisy León Perez talked to me about heading the *Hermanos Zais* Committee for Defense of the Revolution in Havana. In that city, I also chatted with Jesus Hernándes Montalvo who was both president of the *Consejo Popular* in his Havana district and deputy to the *Asamblea Nacional*. I obtained information regarding Birthing Project U.S.A.'s use of Cuban experiences from interviews with its director Kathryn Hall-Trujillo, and its medical director Dr. Sarpoma Sefa-Boakye, a graduate of ELAM. The person I most frequently interviewed was Dr. Julio López Benítez, who provided me with insights into virtually every stage of Cuba's medical development as well as his experiences in South Africa. Cuban journalist Hedelberto López Blanch granted me numerous personal interviews and also organized interviews with others over several years, drove me to many of those interviews, and presented me with a copy of his valuable work, *Historias Secretas de Médicos Cubanos*.

Though my Spanish is fluent enough for me to express my ideas and formulate questions, I fail to capture all the subtleties of rapid speech. For that reason, I am highly grateful to Rebecca Fitz for translating the responses in most of the interviews. Exceptions are the interview with Dr. Piñeiro, translated by Emily Brown, and my exchanges with Dr. Martínez, in which the late Dr. Angel Chang helped me. Finally, Ivan Angulo Torres facilitated my communication with medical staff in Peru.

I deeply appreciate Candace Wolf's making available her interviews with Dr. José Gilberto Fleites Batista, who lived through the Cuban revolution, and his son Dr. Gilberto Fleites Gonzalez, whom I quote extensively. Several staff members at ELAM supported my efforts by providing general information about the school, statistical data regarding students, explanations about how ELAM relates to the Cuban medical system, and help in contacting international students. They include the late ELAM rector, Juan Carrizo, Director of International Relations Nancy Remón Sánchez, General Secretary of Project ELAM Wuilmaris Pérez Torres, Assistant Professor of MGI Dr. Raul Jorge Miranda, and Professor Delfín Marrero.

Just before the March Against Homophobia in Cienfuegos, my wife, Barbara Chicherio, met Mariela Castro, director of the National Sex Education Center. This was during a tour organized by the Medical Education Cooperation with Cuba (MEDICC), which works to enhance cooperation between the United States, Cuba, and health advocates globally. Particularly helpful in providing insights into Cuban medicine during this trip were MEDICC coordinator Anna Dorman, MEDICC translator Georgina "Yoyi" Gómez Tablo, and MEDICC medical consultant Maricela Torres Esperón.

Conner Gorry, who is senior editor of *MEDICC Review*, an English-language peer-reviewed journal focusing on Cuban medicine, has discussed many aspects of Cuban health care with me and provided feedback on drafts of some of my articles. I also thank Daniel Hellinger, Steve Brouwer, Linda M. Whiteford, John M. Kirk, and Joan Roelofs for reading and commenting on early versions of many articles appearing in this book. Publication of some of the chapters as articles in *Monthly Review* was made possible by its staff, including Michael D. Yates, Colin Vanderburg, Spencer Sunshine, Susie Day, Camila Valle, and Chris Gilbert. Michael Albert and Lydia Sargent have encouraged my efforts by printing early versions of some material appearing here in *Z Magazine*.

PERMISSIONS

I thank the publications below for generously permitting me to publish edited versions of essays first appearing in them. Several chapters of this book are edited versions of articles that appeared previously in *Monthly Review* (*MR*). They include the following:

- Chapter 1, "The Three Thousand Who Stayed," *MR* 68/1 (May 2016), 43–56;
- Chapter 2, "Birth of the Cuban Polyclinic," *MR* 70/2 (June 2018), 21–32;
- Chapter 3, "Cuba's First Military Doctors," *MR* 70/6 (November 2018), 46–62;
- Chapter 7, "ELAM: The Latin American School of Medicine," *MR* 62/10 (March 2011), 50–62;
- Chapter 9, "Cuba: The New Global Medicine," *MR* 64/4 (September 2012), 37–46;
- Chapter 11, "Cuba's Medical Mission," *MR* 67/9 (February 2016), 54–61.
- A recently published article in the Cuban journal *Revista Cubana de Salud Pública* provides annual data on the number of doctors practicing medicine and leaving the island during the first decade following the revolution. Since that article provides more up-to-date figures than those used for the *MR* article (70/2, June 2018), "Birth of the Cuban Polyclinic," Table 1 in chapter 2, is based on its data.
- Chapter 8, "Thirteen Faces of ELAM," is an edited version of an article that previously appeared in *Z Magazine* 23/11 (November 2010), 37–41.

- Chapter 10, "Challenges of the Twenty-First Century," includes edited versions of four brief articles. They include the following:
- "Revolutionary Doctors in Venezuela" was originally published as a review of Steve Brouwer's *Revolutionary Doctors: How Venezuela and Cuba Are Changing the World's Conceptualization of Health Care* (New York: Monthly Review Press, 2011) in *Z Magazine* (October 2011), 44–45;
- "Marching Against Homophobia" originally appeared in *Links International Journal of Socialist Renewal*, May 28, 2012, http://links.org.au/node/2884;
- "Combating Dengue Fever" originally appeared in *Black Agenda Report*, February 14, 2012, http://blackagendareport.com/content/med-school-classes-cancelled-havana;
- "Lessons of the Cuban Health Care Model" was originally published in *Black Agenda Report*, December 12, 2012, http://blackagendareport.com/content/why-cuba%E2%80%99s-health-care-system-best-model- poor-countries.

Portions that are original publications for this work include:
- Chapter 4, "From *Policlínico Comunitarios* to Family Medicine";
- Chapter 5, "Cuban Doctors in Angola";
- Chapter 6, "A Time of the Unexpected"; and,
- Chapter 12, "Medicine in Cuba and the United States."

FINAL THANKS

This work would never have been completed without the continued support of two people close to me. The decision of my daughter, Rebecca Vera Fitz, to go to medical school in Cuba altered the direction of my life. As I became intrigued with Cuban medicine, she encouraged me to make trips to the island and introduced me to several of her ELAM classmates. She also guided me to sites in Cuba that I never knew existed and sent many photos, all the while providing me with insights into Cuban culture and translating countless interviews, conversations, and correspondence.

As we learned about the Cuban revolution's extraordinary accomplishments, my wife, Barbara Chicherio, and I discussed every observation either of us had. She aided me in conceptualizing how what happens in Cuba fits into a global environmental framework and encouraged me in my efforts to give voice to the island's achievements. She also read and edited every article before publication and generously tolerated my neglect of social obligations.

— 1 —

THE THREE THOUSAND WHO STAYED

Stories of Cuban medical accomplishments often note that half of the country's roughly six thousand doctors had left within a few years of the revolution. But just as professionals were forsaking their homeland en masse for the comforts of Miami, over three thousand doctors chose to stay. Why did they remain? More important, with the number of patients per doctor now almost doubled, how did they face the daunting task of transforming medicine? In addition to treating patients, their goals included expanding medical care to rural regions; increasing medical education to replace doctors who had left; making care preventive, community-oriented, and focused on tropical diseases; and redesigning a fractured and non-cohesive health system. Exploring changes during this transformative period in Cuban health care requires examining sources available in Cuba, as well as studying oral histories of Cuban physicians who lived during the revolution.

Before 1959, Cuba experienced three medical revolutions. Early "care" had been primitive. Despite the rhetoric of the Spanish invaders, there is no evidence that they brought techniques superior to that of the native Siboney and African folk healers.[1] The first medical revolution (1790–1830) occurred amid brutality against slaves—an early "safety device" being overseers' use of machetes to cut off the hands of slaves caught in rollers. Such events were not uncommon among those forced to work 20 hours per day. The revolution was led by Tomás Romay y Chacón (1764–1849), who introduced smallpox vaccination to Cuba, promoted public sanitation, and advocated medical treatment for slaves. Romay provided Cuban practitioners with an intellectual alternative to blind adherence to Spanish traditions.

The second medical revolution (1898–1922) followed a wave of Cuban doctors deserting their patients, as would happen again following the 1959 upheaval. At this earlier time, doctors fled the countryside to the safety of the cities, during the country's two wars for independence (1868–1878 and 1895–1898). In their absence, disease, already rampant, ravaged the island. Of the 200,000 troops Spain sent to Cuba during the second war, 704 died in battle, 8,164 died of wounds, and 53,000 perished from disease, the most virulent killer being yellow fever, which claimed 13,000 lives. Though Carlos J. Finlay, a leader of the second medical revolution, had discovered the mechanism for the transmission of yellow fever as early as 1881, his research was ridiculed by medical professionals in Cuba, Spain, and the United States, and his findings were not implemented until 1900. A year later, Cuba was free of the disease. Along with the discovery of mosquitos as vectors for malaria and yellow fever, the second medical revolution was known for its emphasis on microbiology and immunology. As Ross Danielson summarizes in his history of Cuban medicine: "The second medical revolution was the completion of the first. Scientific method, gaining superiority as an intellectual device in the first period, yielded convincing practical technology only in the second."[2]

The third medical revolution (1925–1945) was characterized less by new discoveries than heightened awareness. A split within the medical community widened as it became increasingly clear that any resolution of Cuba's medical problems would require focusing on the needs of the rural population, preventive medicine through inexpensive services, and application of new knowledge of tropical medicine and parasitology.[3] It was during this period, in 1925, that the country's first national physicians' organization appeared, the Cuban Medical Federation (FMC). That year also saw the founding of the Cuban Confederation of Workers and the Cuban Communist Party (CCP).[4]

Within four years, the FMC saw the formation of two internal political organizations: Renovación, which pushed for higher physician wages and better university training, and Unión Federativa (UF), which represented doctors in larger private medical organizations. In 1932 Renovación split into two further factions, Reformista and Ala Izquierda (Left Wing). By 1938, the FMC platform called for "pharmaceutical controls, workers' accident protection, a minimum wage scale for physicians, prohibition of multiple positions, institutionalization of the sanitary career, improved hospitals, school health, sanitary provisions for the poor . . . [and] a physicians' retirement plan."[5] Though its program reflected the views of Ala Izquierda, the FMC's leadership remained under the control of the more conservative UF. Increased factionalism produced another, more leftist party, Acción Inmediata (AcIn), and a right-wing party, Ortodoxos, which called for dropping the demand that doctors not hold multiple positions (which made some rich and others under- or unemployed).[6]

Divisions among doctors intensified. AcIn won leadership of the Havana Medical College in 1941, but this leftist victory was reversed when a thousand doctors came to vote in 1942. That same year, however, AcIn won national leadership in the FMC, and in 1943 won again in the Havana Medical College. CCP members held leadership positions in the FMC from 1943 until the 1959 revolution. In 1951, doctors repeated calls for better organization of hospitals, minimum salaries, regulation of specialties, and modern medical standards. Above all, a deep concern for the lack of adequate rural health care defined the third medical revolution.

The three medical revolutions saw "mutualism" grow from a minor footnote to a major chapter in Cuban health care. Cuban historians describe mutualism as "a form of self-financed assistance" whereby a monthly payment covered treatment, hospitalization, and medications.[7] The first mutualist plan was offered four hundred years before the revolution when, in 1559, a Spanish physician proposed a plan for medical care in exchange for a regular fee. Over the centuries, mutualism grew into contradictory subgroupings catering to Spanish immigrants, commercial associations, or unionized workers. Private fee-for-service care existed at the same time. A common complaint was that mutualist doctors would recommend private doctors for services not covered by the mutualist plan; then the two physicians would split the fees. Nevertheless, mutualist clinics fostered a collective attitude toward medical work, which would become critical after the 1959 revolution. Alongside mutualism and fee-for-service care was the state medical system, which provided limited care to the poor. On the eve of the 1959 revolution there were abundant, overlapping medical systems in the cities but rife negligence in rural Cuba. Of 456 health institutions during 1956, 42.8 percent were private or mutualist. Of these, 52 percent were in Havana.

MEDICAL CARE TRANSFORMED

Ten years after the revolution, Fidel Castro described the enormity of the health care problems that confronted Cuba in January 1959:

> The absence of a national public health plan; semi-official and private services that were better than those provided by the government; an orientation toward curative medicine; abandonment of rural and some urban areas; individual medicine; mercantilism; competition between private services; administrative centralization with a public unaware of treatments that could benefit them.[8]

In addition, there was no reliable data on health indicators, an insufficient number of doctors and dentists being trained, and severe underfunding for the few existing research facilities. The pharmacy industry was 70 percent foreign-controlled and created many products lacking treatment value. Only 10 percent of children were covered by specialized pediatric care. Vaccination programs were unavailable.[9]

When he was eighty-seven years old, Dr. José Gilberto Fleites Batista recalled the revolutionary epoch to Candace Wolf: "Before the Revolution, there were big hospitals only in the capital, in big cities, but not in rural areas, in the countryside and in the Sierra."[10] The physician-to-inhabitant ratio was 1 to 248 in Havana and 1 to 2,608 in the eastern provinces. Medical education was largely theoretical, offering little hands-on experience. There were not enough teaching hospitals, and education was oriented to making money. Dr. Julio López Benítez completed his specialty in pediatric nephrology in 1960, shortly after Havana's medical school reopened following the revolution. He remembers that "some were in medicine as a business. In Calixto-García Hospital, three hundred professors charged their patients."[11]

The principal health care task during the first five years of the revolution was creating services. In 1959, priority went to hospital construction. By 1963, the revolutionary government had established 122 rural centers and forty-two rural hospitals, with 1,155 beds, 322 doctors, and 49 dentists. In order to accomplish the primary task, it was necessary to bring cohesion to the disjointed medical system. On January 22, 1960, Law 717 created the Ministerio de Salud Pública (Ministry of Public Health, or MINSAP) and Law 723 established Rural Health Services.[12] As MINSAP consolidated and extended state services, it had an ambivalent attitude toward mutualism, which was based on privately owned services. Nevertheless, it would have been a serious blunder to attempt to abolish mutualist clinics during the upheavals following the revolution. Widespread mutualist services provided a cushion for the effects of doctors' abandoning private practice as they left the island. This lessened the pressure on public services as they expanded and reorganized. As time went by, contradictions within mutualism intensified as its members realized that its services were inconsistent and health care could be obtained at no cost through state clinics. Instead of attacking the system, MINSAP developed a 1963 report describing how to consolidate and rationalize mutualism.

Revolutionary changes cannot be made by legislative decree alone.

They require the type of mobilization campaigns that swept Cuba. There were efforts to end unemployment, increase the salary of 350,000 sugarcane workers, implement a pension system, end discrimination in access to beaches, build 10,000 new classrooms, and send 3,000 teachers to rural areas. A new rationing system ensured equitable distribution of food and consumer goods. Pointing to the need for preventive care, it focused on pregnant women, undernourished infants, and children with chronic illnesses.

The literacy campaign was the best known of these mobilization efforts. In 1953, 23.6 percent of the Cuban population was illiterate (41.7 percent in rural areas). In a single year, more than 707,000 people were taught to read and write. Within a few years, the campaign brought illiteracy down to zero. These early campaigns were launched at a time when Batista supporters still roamed the countryside. Fleites recalls: "Thousands of students went into the countryside to teach the people how to read and write. It was a beautiful campaign, but it came with a harsh price. The counterrevolutionaries assassinated some of these idealistic students."

Medical and education campaigns were thus essential components of a much broader social transformation. In 1960, Law 723 required medical graduates to spend a year in rural service. By 1963, 1,500 doctors and fifty dentists had served in rural Cuba. In February 1960, the first group of 357 doctors went to areas where there had previously been no doctors. Many had to stay in the homes of *campesinos*, peasant farmers. They found people so much in need that initially they could provide only curative, rather than preventive, medicine. Efforts to implement preventive medicine went forward, however, and by the end of 1960 doctors had given twice as many DPT vaccines (for diphtheria, pertussis, and tetanus) as had been provided during the five years previous to the revolution.

The anti-malaria campaign began in 1961. The next year saw the first national campaign to vaccinate against polio, a clean water campaign, gastroenteritis control, and a major program to improve medical staff training. There was even an anti-rabies campaign for street dogs. MINSAP developed fifteen goals for the years 1962 to

1965 that focused on "infant mortality, vaccinations, pregnant women, transmissible diseases, infectious diseases, preventive medicine, worker health, and goals for administering these and recording statistics systematically."[13] Simultaneously, it improved plans for hurricane disaster relief and cut the price of eyeglasses and medications by 50 percent.

NEW DOCTORS, NEW EDUCATION

The wave of revolutionary fervor sweeping through the island took a distinctive form in medical school education. Batista had responded to protests by closing the University of Havana, including its medical school, from 1957 to 1958. When the school reopened in 1959, there was a new approach to education. Dr. Enzo Dueñas Gómez had a specialty in pediatric neonatology and was in the first class to graduate after the revolution. He told me how, following the revolution, "the culture of teaching changed. In the classical medical education before 1959, students could go to class if they felt like it and they received little practical experience. This is why they could skip class. After the revolution, students had to get to class for practical experience and go to rural areas."[14]

Dr. Felipe Cárdenas Gonzáles graduated in 1962 with a specialty in pediatric cardiac surgery. He observed a new way of recruiting students: "We created a new culture of revolutionary medicine. The professors of medicine who stayed went out looking for good students who could become doctors."[15] Inspired by free tuition, many of the new students came from working-class backgrounds. Once enrolled, they found a plethora of revolutionary organizations. Incoming students were required to take classes focusing on rural and tropical medicine as well as preclinical sciences. For the first time, the medical school taught biochemistry. Hospital internships were made a prerequisite for graduation. Before 1959, a short course on social medicine was offered in the last year, after students had already formed their clinical perspectives. After 1959, social medicine was included in each year's curriculum.

Student and government involvement was reforming old systems of faculty control over education. On July 29, 1960, the medical faculty was evenly divided when it met to discuss a proposed Superior Governing Board for the university. A month later, in August 1960, only nineteen professors remained in the medical school—the only one in Cuba. They formed a nucleus of young, competent doctors who took on monumental responsibilities to sustain the medical training system.

To accommodate more students, the number of teaching hospitals increased from four to seven, and new medical schools opened in Las Villas and Santiago de Cuba. Students and doctors adjusted to the strenuous demands of the revolution. "No one rested during those years," Cárdenas remembers. "We worked as hard as we needed to. I did *guardia* for 24 hours and then I did surgery and then I had to study and write a work-up for new students." MINSAP contracted medical instructors from twenty-six countries: 120 arrived in 1964 and 92 in 1965. Most came from Argentina, Mexico, and Ecuador. Others were from Bulgaria, the Soviet Union, Czechoslovakia, and Hungary.

Ross Danielson writes: "Other responses by the university to the flight of physicians included a reduction of the pre-internship period from 6 to 4 years, and from 4 to 3 years in dentistry."[16] I asked four physicians—Dueñas, López Benítez, Cárdenas, and Mena—how the shortened period affected teaching, and all denied that such a process had happened. López Benítez was emphatic: "I participated in developing the curriculum for fourteen educational plans, beginning in 1963, and we never had fewer than six years of study."[17] Though shortening the required period of medical study might seem like an efficient crash course to train more doctors, it appears unlikely that it was ever done. The first five years of revolution had transformed the culture of medicine and provided care to those who had never received it, but doctor-to-patient ratios had not improved.

"Wherever the Revolution Needs Me"

The new government, and particularly Fidel, received a tremendous response to calls for revolutionary commitments. Fleites's enthusiasm was born from dislike of the Batista regime:

> I sympathized with the revolutionaries, but I lived outside of that. My world consisted of operating on my patients and taking care of my family. The only time that the revolution and the operating room came together for me was when I hid a young man—a wounded revolutionary fighter who was running from Batista's police. He arrived in the emergency room while I was an intern at the Calixto García Hospital and I hid him there from the police who would have tortured or killed him. But I will tell you that the triumph of the Revolution was a great moment for all of us.[18]

Even before the government required rural medical service, on November 29, 1959, medical students assembled to pledge their willingness to go to provincial Cuba. Soon after López Benítez graduated from medical school, he said, "a friend asked me why doctors were being sent to Santiago when there were not enough in Havana and I said that there were even fewer in Santiago. We're all Cubans."

As Cuban society polarized, students were entering medical school with the expectation that they would be trained not for personal gain but according to the needs of society. Renouncing private practice, students often commented that they would go "wherever the revolution needs me." By 1963, it was very clear to those entering medical school that they were different from earlier generations of students.

Eagerness to go to the countryside likewise caught fire with practicing physicians. Fleites was profoundly affected by his chat with the new minister of health: "That minister knew me and he talked to me about going with them. They needed many physicians to go to various places in the Sierra Maestra, to provide care for the peasants. And I said 'Yes, I will go!'" López Benítez observed that "Fidel had a huge influence after the literacy campaign. He asked for people to study medicine and many who answered the call were teenagers." One of those teenagers was Dr. Oscar Mena Hector, who spoke to me when he was sixty-two. He heard Fidel's call when he was in middle school. He took the science entrance exams for medical school when he was fourteen years old. He did not pass then, but he did in 1970 and became a doctor in 1976. Medical campaigns in rural Cuba deeply affected those who participated. Fleites "will always remember the particular case of a dehydrated little boy. We gave him intravenous infusions because he had diarrhea. I remember that boy well because he would have died of dehydration if we hadn't been there."

MEDICAL INTERNATIONALISM

Cuba's medical system interacted with other countries in many ways. As early as April 1961, Cuba signed a cooperation agreement with Czechoslovakia. The next year it sent technicians to Bulgaria to study preventive medicine. East Germany made an agreement in 1964 to send orthopedic supplies. Cuba also sent doctors abroad. In March 1960, only fifteen months after the revolution, an earthquake hit Chile, and Cuba sent a small number of doctors for a brief period. The next year Cuba sent arms to Algerians fighting for independence from France. The boat returned with seventy-six injured Algerians and twenty child refugees.

A medical brigade sent to Algeria in 1963 had fifty-five Cubans, including twenty-nine doctors. There were forty-three men and twelve women. Details of this mission were not widely known until Hedelberto López Blanch published *Historias Secretas de Médicos Cubanos* (Secret Stories of Cuban Doctors), a collection of oral histories of Cuban medical workers serving in Africa in the 1960s and 1970s.[19] One of the doctors going to Algeria was Dr. Sara Perelló, who was eighty-four years old when interviewed by López Blanch. She had just graduated with a specialty in pediatrics. Her mother had heard Fidel saying that the flight of doctors to France left Algerians even worse off than Cubans: "There are 4 million more Algerians than Cubans but they have only a third of the doctors we do."[20] After her mother came home and told her that she needed to help them, Perelló went to MINSAP to volunteer. She was worried about leaving because her elderly mother was suffering from Parkinson's disease. Her mother responded that Sara's sister and husband would help her as would the government: "Now the thing to do is go forward and don't worry about your mother, who will be well taken care of."[21]

When Dr. Pablo Resik Habib was seventy-six years old, he told López Blanch that he was chosen to head the Algerian mission largely because of his Arab heritage. He had worked as an anesthesiologist, first in a hospital and then in a mutualist clinic. He left his three-month-old daughter in the care of his wife, who supported the international efforts. Brigade members were promised a small stipend, with their salaries going to their families. Resik described the precarious plunge into Cuba's first international mission: "We found ourselves in an Arabic country, Muslim, with habits, customs and cultures very different from ours."[22]

Dr. Zoila Italia Suárez would have completed her pediatric specialty, but due to Batista's closure of the university, her graduation was delayed until 1960. She went immediately to Granma province for her rural services. Her recruitment to the Algerian brigade exemplifies the transition from campaigns to end the rural-urban dichotomy within Cuba to medical internationalism. Her initial willingness to leave Havana for rural Cuba easily transformed into a willingness to help meet medical needs in Africa. Italia emphasized that language was her main problem. During treatment she would have one translator for Arabic to French and a second for French to Spanish. When one woman brought in a child but spoke a form of Arabic that the translator did not understand, the mother took her hand and placed it on her son's abdomen. Upon feeling a tumor, she sent him to the hospital immediately. She learned to diagnose based on where the mother touched the child or if she imitated sneezing or coughing.

The mission taught staff valuable medical experiences. Italia witnessed "many sicknesses that were rare or nonexistent in Cuba. I saw a lot of tuberculosis, malnutrition, malaria, parasitic diseases and bacterial infections. . . . In Constantina, a military hospital was completely empty because the French doctors had left."[23] Ernesto "Che" Guevara left a deep mark on this formative mission. Italia recalled:

"Che visited us when we had only been in Algeria a month. He asked if we were having any difficulties and how we were able to interact with patients without knowing their language. Che only spent a few hours with us; but we were distributed in various provinces and he went throughout the country."[24] Dr. Perelló reminisced, "One afternoon we were told that Che would meet us the next morning at 7 a.m. We didn't think that would happen because no one travels at night in Algeria. But when we arrived at the government house on April 13, 1963, Che was waiting for us at the door." Che impressed her as serious to the point of being ascetic: "Che told us to forget the greenery and palm trees of Cuba and dedicate ourselves to our work."[25] Algerian experiences left Cubans with stories that would inspire medical students for decades. Resik emphasized, "I received much more from this mission than I gave to it. . . . I am proud to have been one of the pioneers of this enormous example that the small island of the Caribbean has given to the world."[26]

THOSE WHO LEFT

Many Cuban doctors had no desire to go to the provinces, much less to the Algerian desert. Multiple waves of doctors left Cuba after the revolution. The first accompanied the huge changes in health care delivery during the first couple of years. Many were owners of private clinics, directors of mutualist centers, and doctors who enjoyed high incomes from private practice. The second wave was provoked by the April 1961 Bay of Pigs invasion and the October 1962 missile crisis. López Benítez pointed out that "in William Soler Hospital there were fifty-nine doctors. In one day in February 1961, twenty-six left. This was a month or so before the Bay of Pigs. They must have known that it would happen and left before."

Many departed with the advent of rural service, which would take them to locations lacking the comforts of Havana. Cárdenas stated: "It was similar to Brazil where many doctors do not want to go to areas where they are most needed." He added, "Most of the doctors who left were not rich but identified with them." The literacy, medical, and other campaigns that brought contact with Cuba's poor, working, and farming classes were an affront to middle-class lifestyles. It went beyond the disruption of medical school—when Batista closed the university during the years 1957 to 1958, there was no great exodus of medical faculty. Dueñas suggested, "They knew that doors were open to them in the United States. Many doctors went to Miami not because they were counterrevolutionaries but because they could have so many things in the United States."

I asked four doctors—López Benítez, Cárdenas, Dueñas, and Mena—if the difference between those who left and stayed was primarily a generation gap, and they all replied no, age had nothing to do with it. They also agreed that it was not possible to know how a doctor would react to the revolution based on his wealth. "Roberto Guerra was a well-known rich surgeon," Dueñas pointed out. "He was very charismatic, with no children but a movie star lover. He was the first to give up his private practice and donated his clinic to the revolution so that it could be used for teaching." "Dr. José Resno Albara renounced his millions of dollars and helped found the new revolutionary medicine," López Benítez added. "Some doctors supported the revolution after it happened, but some had been revolutionaries." I asked, "Does this mean that you could not know before 1959 who would help and who would not?"—and heard an emphatic "Yes!"

Although it would be an overstatement to imply that there was no relationship between pre- and post-revolution attitudes of doctors, it would likewise be an overstatement to suggest that actions before 1959 could always predict a doctor's loyalties afterward. Certainly some who were enthralled by the July 26 Movement became dismayed once they saw that the revolution actually implemented its ideas (rather than abandoning them, as in so many other successful Latin American revolutions). Conversely, many who had initially remained aloof from the struggle—perhaps believing that Cuba could never undergo a genuine transformation—later threw themselves into the struggle once underway. The defining contrast between the doctors who stayed and those who left was their attitude toward revolution as it actually took shape: whether they were enraptured or repulsed by the changes unfolding before them.

RACE AND THE MEDICAL REVOLUTION

Cubans of African descent were concentrated in the rural eastern part of the island, which is closer to Haiti and where Santiago de Cuba is the largest city. It is hard to overstate the importance of the 1959 revolution, which ushered in the most significant changes in the lives of black Cubans since the abolition of slavery. Calls to serve in rural areas and eastern provinces were equivalent to appeals to fight structural racism. These shifts inspired López Benítez to volunteer for service: "I was doing genetic research as a pediatrician when they told me that children were dying in Santiago and that I needed to get there; so I went to Santiago in the early '60s for a three-month rotation."

Pre-revolutionary racism had not been subtle or limited, but rather open and uncompromising. López Benítez described one hospital that "claimed that it was dedicated to religious goals; but it only accepted white patients and would not accept black patients." Mena's family knew racism well. His cousin José Villena "studied medicine but was poor and had to sell tomatoes to buy books. He passed all his courses, but after his last exam learned that he would not become a doctor because he was black." Studies culminated in a tribunal exam, and one examining physician refused to pass black students. "Two years later, in 1959, he passed his exams and became a doctor." José Villena practiced internal medicine in Camaguey until his death.

The pre-revolutionary period was not without anti-racist efforts in health care, however. In 1938 the communist-led Transport Workers Union began a mutualist health plan with a clinic for its workers, the Centro Benéfico. After five years, it offered the plan to other workers and enrolled 25,000 by 1959. "*The* Centro Benéfico," writes Ross Danielson, "*was the only mutualist clinic which served a substantial number of nonwhite Cubans and served them without discrimination or segregation*" (italics in original).[27] The outpouring of medical teams to poor urban communities, rural areas, and the eastern part of the island with coordination by the revolutionary government occurred at the same time that U.S. civil rights demonstrators were being beaten by police and attacked by dogs for demanding the right to sit at "whites-only" lunch counters. This contrast was not lost on Cubans or many in the United States.

A New Consciousness

The central contradiction facing revolutionary medicine was how to do much more with much less while also thinking and planning deeper than ever before. Writing twenty years after the revolution, Roberto Capote Mir summarized the period's early accomplishments: creating a unified health system; increasing hospital beds and health care facilities, especially in rural and eastern Cuba; increasing every category of health care worker; and attaining "active participation by the masses in the solution of health care problems."[28] Of the many organizations created at the time, by far the most important for medicine were the Committees for Defense of the Revolution (CDRs), organized in 1960 to guard against the counterrevolution. CDRs participated in multiple health campaigns, and, after 1962, were responsible for polio immunization.

In a different political climate doctors became different people. "When I started my medical career," López Benítez told me, "I thought that if a child died of hunger it was not my problem as a doctor. But now I understand that it is my problem." Dr. Cárdenas was no less affected:

> At the beginning people were for or against the revolution in a very theoretical way, but I became married to the revolution. There was a vaccination campaign in Realengo 18 [in Guantánamo]. Patients had to come by foot and a woman brought a child who had gastroenteritis. His father had to walk for three hours every day to see him and I told him he could stay home because his son could leave in two days. The father would

not leave because he said four other sons had died. This changed my life forever.

As physicians began to act as medical "cadres," they perceived themselves as embedded in a broader political agenda. A medical school graduate "could not fail to see his own efforts as only one part of a set of health-related measures: land reform, new roads, improved agricultural methods, schools, literacy programs, improved diet, and an end to seasonal unemployment."[29]

The imperative to serve the underserved became the guiding idea of medicine in Cuba. As Karl Marx wrote: "Theory becomes a material force when it grips the masses."[30] The sheer desire of isolated physicians to provide care at no cost to impoverished Cubans could not on its own change medicine, any more than could a government attempting to create a new medical system by decree, if isolated from the mood of the country. But in a country where thousands of doctors had struggled for decades to create equitable health care, a revolutionary government that reflected that awareness could unite those struggles and reshape medicine.

The consciousness of the three thousand who stayed became the "material force" in the production of Cuban health care, as much a material force as the manufacture of pharmaceuticals or the construction of hospitals. Medicine was affected by that consciousness at least as much as Cuban dentistry was affected by the newly developed high-speed drills that Fidel acquired as ransom from the United States for the return of mercenaries captured after the Bay of Pigs invasion.

Still unanswered, however, was whether this new medical consciousness would be powerful enough to overcome new challenges. The need for basic services was so severe that meeting it required building physical facilities and focusing on specific illnesses and health problems. The relationship of health care institutions to the communities they served remained much the same. Though the municipal polyclinic, begun in 1962, offered a new orientation, the atmosphere of crisis prevented this paradigm shift from expanding.[31] The question remained: Once the delivery of services improved, would the medical field be able to plan and enact fundamental changes in the way health care was delivered?

Another dark cloud hung over medicine: infant mortality increased during the first few years of the revolution.[32] It is likely that a portion of the increase was attributable to more accurate statistics. Some infant deaths that would not have been tabulated before 1959 were recorded after the revolution. The revolution was doing everything humanly possible to provide vaccinations and other pediatric services, but the flight of doctors took its toll. Schools were working sleeplessly to expand every type of medical training, and doctors were much more evenly distributed throughout the island. Yet by the end of 1963, there was still a lower doctor-to-patient ratio than there had been in January 1959. The question remained: Would new students be able to continue such an intense pace and increase their numbers through the coming years?

Though medical accomplishments were felt throughout the island, the trip of fifty-five medical staff to Algeria was not well publicized. Five years after the revolution, no one knew what their impact would be. Would the efforts in health care later be viewed as a waste of desperately needed resources? Or would the experiences gained from the Algerian mission combine with medical approaches that were still embryonic within Cuba, and this marriage transform revolutionary dreams into a material force favoring the production of a new global medicine?

— 2 —

BIRTH OF THE CUBAN POLYCLINIC

During the 1960s, Cuban medicine experienced changes as tumultuous as the civil rights and antiwar protests in the United States. While activists, workers, and students in Western Europe and the United States confronted existing institutions of capitalism and imperialism, Cuba faced the even greater challenge of building a new society.

The tasks of Cuban medicine differed sharply between the first and the second halves of the revolution's initial decade. The years 1959 to 1964 were dedicated to overcoming the crisis of care delivery, as half of the island's physicians fled. It was during the second half of the decade (1964–69) that Cuba began redesigning medicine as an integrated system. The resulting reconceptualization of health care, which put the area polyclinic at the center of medical care, created a model for poor countries that changed medicine ever after.

THE *POLICLÍNICO INTEGRAL*

When the revolutionary government took power in 1959, millions of Cubans were without medical care. The revolution put enormous energy into building new facilities and expanding services. Nowhere was the crisis more severe than among the island's rural and black population.[1]

The revolution had inherited a patchwork of unintegrated, overlapping medical structures, including private fee-for-service practices, public assistance for the poor, a few large medical plans, and many small plans.[2] These rarely offered preventive medicine and never a complete range of treatment, requiring patients to go from one provider to another (if another was even available). Though the second half-decade of the revolution continued to expand care, it focused on reorganizing the disjointed medical system it had inherited.

Accounts of Cuban medicine during the 1960s can be confusing. Some emphasize the increase in the number of polyclinics without noting their metamorphosis in the middle of the decade.[3] The term "polyclinic" (*policlínico*) generally refers to a medical facility offering outpatient services. José Ruíz Hernández clarifies what happened in the Cuban system of *policlínicos*: in August 1961, the Ministry of Public Health (MINSAP) began a study in Marianao (a town of 45,000) that sought to unify preventive and curative medicine. In May 1964 it became the first *policlínico integral* in Cuba.[4] The next year, MINSAP began to spread the *policlínico integral* model throughout Cuba, making it "the point of departure for all health planning."[5]

How did the *policlínico integral* differ from earlier *policlínicos*, and why was it so central to creating the new medicine? MINSAP's plan addressed existing shortcomings by consolidating services. Staff at the new polyclinics would include at least a general practice physician, nurse, pediatrician, OB/GYN, and social worker.[6] Dentistry was also brought on board, and nurses and social workers made house calls.[7] Staff extended services to workplaces, schools, and communities. Outreach included health campaigns such as mass vaccination programs and efforts to control malaria and dengue.

Vaccination began shortly after the revolution, but the *policlínico integral* structure vastly increased its effectiveness. In 1962, 80 percent of all Cuban children under fifteen were vaccinated against polio in eleven days. In 1970, it took just one day for the same national effort.[8] Malaria was eradicated in 1967, as was diphtheria by 1971.[9]

Clinic staff coordinated primary care programs (maternal and child care, adult medical care, and dentistry) as well as public health, including control of infectious diseases, environmental services, food safety, school health, and occupational and labor medicine.[10] The *policlínicos integrales* were designed to integrate medical services in multiple ways. In addition to combining preventive and curative medicine, they provided a full range of services at a single location, coordinated community campaigns, and offered social as well as medical services. Most important, they provided a single point of entry into the system, allowing for a complete record of patients' medical histories and making them key to the transformation of health care.

It cannot be overemphasized that these advances in medical care could only have succeeded through the massive changes in Cuban society that began immediately after the revolution and continued during the ensuing decade. The best known was the literacy campaign of 1961, but other programs addressed racial discrimination, land reform, agricultural salaries, farming methods, improved diet, pensions, new roads, new classrooms, housing, piped water, and urban–rural differences. The redesign of medical services was thus hardly an isolated process—it was an essential component of remaking Cuba.

Mutualism Withers Away

The second half of the decade saw continued efforts to build up the number of medical staff and assign them to rural and poor urban areas. By 1969, twenty nursing schools had been opened on the island.[11] The number of nurses climbed from 2,500 in 1958 to more than 4,300 in 1968.[12] Similar pushes were made to augment the number of auxiliary nurses, X-ray technicians, laboratory technicians, sanitarians, and dental assistants. Always attentive to alternative medicine, Cubans also integrated healers (*curanderos*) into the health system, and MINSAP provided them with salaries and training as auxiliary personnel.[13] As dentists were absorbed by the polyclinics, their numbers more than quadrupled, from 250 in 1958 to 1,081 in 1967.[14]

Though the first plan for a comprehensive national health service was developed in 1961 and implemented the next year, it was significantly revised in 1965.[15] The new version sought to alter the structure of the medical system itself, as MINSAP turned its attention to the unbalanced number, proportion, and location of medical facilities. Only around a fifth of Cubans lived in Havana, but the city had more than half of the country's hospital beds. By comparison, the rural Oriente, the eastern part of the island, with a larger black population, was home to 35 percent of all Cubans but had only 15.5 percent of hospital beds.[16] Thus, plans for new beds and doctors were concentrated in the east.

Also problematic were the many rural hospitals with fewer than a hundred beds that could not provide a full range of services. Greater efficiency required an increase in rural polyclinics and concentration of hospitals in cities. The number of hospitals accordingly decreased from 339 in 1958 to 219 in 1969. In the same period, the number of beds per hospital more than doubled, from 83 to 181. The total number of hospital beds increased from 25,170 to 41,027—or, from 3.8 to 5.1 beds per one thousand Cubans.[17]

The polyclinic took on a more central role, as more patients were initially seen at polyclinics, where a physician could refer them to a hospital. The number of health visits doubled between 1965 and 1969, but visits to hospitals dropped from 28 to 19 percent of the total. At the same time, trips to polyclinics went up from 32 to 63 percent of total medical visits.

Clinics changed not only in number but in type. Mutualism, the prevailing model in Cuba for four centuries, was a pre-revolutionary holdover unable to resolve health issues with its scattered array of unconnected services. Nevertheless, it remained immensely popular. A key task of the revolutionary government was to resolve these contradictions. Mutualism broadly resembled insurance, with subscribers paying a monthly fee for hospitalization and medical services. The types of services covered varied widely from plan to plan, and none covered everything. Of 456 Cuban health institutions in 1956, 42.8 percent were private or mutualist.[18] Often owned by rich doctors, these entities were a major barrier to an integrated medical system with facilities that could provide a complete range of services. Unlike the new *policlínicos integrales*, mutualist clinics did not offer preventive medicine, were not adequately linked to hospitals, and did not serve specific geographical areas.

Nevertheless, given the popularity of mutualist clinics, the revolutionary government was wise not to nationalize them outright, as it did with many large, foreign-owned businesses in the early 1960s.[19] Instead, MINSAP created a task force in 1963 "to consolidate and rationalize mutualism."[20] In Havana, mutualist clinics were required to provide comprehensive services, and, after 1967, the mutualism budget was included in the MINSAP budget.[21] As mutualist clinics were required to provide services similar to those of government clinics and ceased to be separately funded their distinct role was withering away. In 1970, mutualist plans stopped accepting new members and charging monthly dues, offering equalized services for members and non-members alike—and thereby ceased to exist.

Private medical practice, while not prohibited, likewise faded away. Though some authors suggest that private practice had ended by 1968 or 1969, Ross Danielson writes that there were still eighty full-time private physicians on the island as late at 1970.[22] By the early 1970s, Cuba had a unified medical system, with a focus on the polyclinic for care delivery and all services guided by MINSAP.

CENTRALIZATION/DECENTRALIZATION

Cuban planners carefully studied health systems in the Soviet bloc, especially that of Czechoslovakia. These systems were often overcentralized, leaving little room for individual initiative by practitioners or local administrators. In response, Cuban officials developed the concept of "centralization/decentralization," which aimed to address such risks by making the *policlínico integral* a unique institution of Cuban medicine.

Shortly after the revolution in August 1959 the government adopted the approach of "normative centralization and executive decentralization." The central administration would set norms or guidelines for health care, but local executives would specify how those guidelines would be put into practice.[23] Centralization increased when the year-old revolution established MINSAP with Law 717 in January 1960, and further increased with a 1966 statute creating ten new research institutes.[24] By 1967, MINSAP was overseeing virtually all professional services. In addition to drafting guidelines and overseeing research, this included budgetary control, supervision of three medical schools, and training programs for a variety of health care staff.[25]

What may be difficult for non-Cubans to grasp is that decentralization increased alongside centralization. As mutualist clinics were drawn into the medical system, MINSAP opened new base clinics and expanded their decision-making power. Whereas certain programs were under vertical control, such as those for tuberculosis, leprosy, and venereal disease, polyclinics were given broad discretion over their implementation, improving efficiency.[26] In general, the period saw a process unifying and standardizing the rapidly expanding system of clinics while decentralizing clinic management and increasing autonomy.

This made a lasting impression on physicians living through those times. Dr. María Luísa Lima recalled that "MINSAP centralized the norms and research. Hospitals and polyclinics decided how to document use of drugs and which antibiotics to use for diseases. Hospitals and polyclinics decided how to do things such as managing their equipment."[27] Dr. Julio López felt the same: "There are norms regarding medical tasks. There is not a straightjacket about how to do things. Hospitals and polyclinics have to decide how to do many things. There must be a balance between working within rules while having a lot of freedom to make decisions."[28]

As the era of polyclinics began, the Cuban government charted a course that would ensure their role as the cornerstone of decentralization: the *policlínicos integrales* would be independent of hospital control. The clinics would be distinct entities answering to MINSAP in each region. Instead of acting as administrative branches of regional hospitals, their position would be equal to that of hospitals within the regional administration of MINSAP.[29]

Clinic independence was a key factor distinguishing Cuba's approach from that of the Soviet bloc countries, as well as from other regionalized medical systems in Latin America, such as Puerto Rico and Chile.[30] Cuban doctors were well aware of this distinction. Dr. Oscar Mena emphasized to me that "the hospital does not give orders to the polyclinic. Polyclinics get orders from the regional administration and MINSAP."[31]

As mentioned, the proportion of health care visits was shifting sharply from hospitals toward polyclinics. This meant that "the polyclinic—predominantly an outpatient facility independent of hospital control—was regarded as the core of the health services system as a whole."[32] Though polyclinics were independent from hospitals, their daily functions were interconnected. Hospitals performed and analyzed lab work for nearby polyclinics, and hospital doctors worked part-time in polyclinics, both as consultants and care providers. Similarly, polyclinic doctors worked for brief shifts in hospitals.[33] By the end of the decade, each of the country's 268 polyclinics provided care to 25,000 to 30,000 Cubans, and each of the thirty-eight regional hospital "centers" was affiliated with an average of seven polyclinics. A larger number of provincial hospital centers provided specialty care.[34]

A subtle but important change that elevated the standing of the *policlínico integral* was the creation of primary care as a specialty, addressing everyday medical problems in clinics. Offering primary care as an option for postgraduate training put these physicians on par with other medical specialists as part of the core staff of *policlínicos integrales*. Other forces further decentralized control into the hands of doctors. Instead of developing into an ossified bureaucracy, MINSAP relied on physicians for many aspects of its redesign.[35] Physicians were also working closely with the military amid sustained threats of invasion and nuclear war.[36]

MOBILIZATION FOR A HEALTH REVOLUTION

Policlínicos integrales thus became the unifying link in the structure and services of the new national medical system, which made clinics independent of hospital control and authorized them to determine how to enact guidelines, create their own specialists, and, most importantly, cover a specific geographic service area for which they became the entry point for all local patients. Yet nothing enhanced their stature more in the eyes of average Cubans or better solidified their position in the decentralization of health services than their role in coordinating health campaigns.

Fidel Castro and his comrades understood that a government could not merely decree that a campaign would occur; the literacy campaign showed that successful campaigns require massive mobilization and public enthusiasm. The *policlínicos integrales* walked the same path, and Fidel took a front-and-center position in the mobilization. He motivated physicians, graduating medical students, and the entire country by reminding them that "public health occupies a prioritized and sacred place in the revolution."[37] He pushed for changes that would accelerate training of medical personnel and rotate professors, instructors, and residents from Havana to new medical schools in Santiago (opened in 1962) and Las Villas (1966). By 1969, doctors were teaching at forty hospitals in Havana alone.[38]

One of Fidel's most important contributions was to show that Cuba could improve on Eastern Europe's concept of community clinics. He believed Cuba needed to create an example of public medicine that could be used by other poor and underdeveloped countries. The USSR donated equipment and 850 beds to the recently built Lenin Hospital in Holguín in 1965. Cuba's "repayment" was to provide medical care in even poorer countries, including Guinea, the Congo, Mali, and Vietnam. International solidarity in public health would be one of Fidel's indelible legacies.[39]

In Eastern Europe, the Red Cross was often central in coordinating public health efforts. But the importance of the Cuban Red Cross was tiny compared to the country's voluntary mass organizations.[40] These included the National Association of Small Farmers, which helped establish the first rural health centers and control tuberculosis; the Federation of Cuban Women, which addressed health education, family nutrition, and maternal and child health; and the

Confederation of Cuban Workers, which focused on safety committees in workplaces and state farms, as well as food safety.[41]

By far the most important of the mass organizations were the Committees for Defense of the Revolution (CDRs), first organized in 1960 to guard against sabotage and attacks from the United States. These provided social networks for neighborhoods and soon became integrally linked to public health efforts.[42] By 1962, the CDRs had almost total responsibility for coordinating polio immunizations, shortening the time needed for national vaccination from eleven days to one after the establishment of *policlínicos integrales*. By 1968, the CDRs had enrolled over a third of the Cuban population.[43] CDRs also took on the task of registering the entire population at *policlínicos integrales*.[44] Since each *policlínico integral* had a defined geographical area, 100 percent enrollment was an achievable goal.[45] Working with *policlínicos integrales*, the CDRs were deeply involved in establishing social and preventive medicine; educating and mobilizing the population to help combat flies and mosquitoes, control infectious diseases, and donate blood; building schools and parks; and cleaning and repairing streets.[46] The latter activities are more closely connected to health care than they may seem: patching potholes is a good way to avoid injury from walking, cycling, or driving over them—and is thus sound preventive medicine.

The director of the local polyclinic was also the chair of the Area Health Commission, which included the CDRs and other mass organizations. Thus the polyclinic was simultaneously linked to hospitals by sharing physicians and to the community through its central role in coordinating health campaigns.[47] Vicente Navarro observes that Latin American scholars often attribute inadequate medical care in poor countries to a simple lack of resources. But the first decade of the Cuban Revolution shows that when limited resources are distributed equitably, medical miracles can happen. Similarly, it seems "unlikely that a redistribution of resources would have occurred without substantial redistribution of the decision-making power."[48] The keys to Cuba's medical revolution were (a) dedication and work by all health care professionals; and (b) a well-guided structure, set forth by

MINSAP; with (c) decentralized implementation of health campaigns by *policlínicos integrals*, in coordination with mass organizations.

LINGERING ISSUES

Despite the achievement of a unified medical system with a single point of patient entry via the decentralized *policlínico integral*, significant issues persisted after the revolution's first decade. Most disturbing was that infant mortality continued to climb. This could have been due to improved recording of deaths, but an official Cuban source accepts the data as correct, attributing the rise to early neonatal death rates.[49] Linda Whiteford and Lawrence Branch agree, noting that "since infant mortality reflects prenatal care and nutrition as well as conditions during and immediately following birth, it is not unusual to see such a pattern as a reflection of social upheaval."[50] Whatever the reason, infant deaths grew from thirty-seven (per thousand live births) in 1965 to forty in 1969.[51]

Another concern was that the fusion of centralization and decentralization was often more bumpy than hoped. Even though many revolutionary doctors took positions in MINSAP or as administrators of medical facilities, conflicts still surfaced between those charged with recreating the medical system and those whose daily work focused on care delivery.[52] Sometimes contention was based on policy. Physician Julio López recalls: "Many doctors and administrators felt like polyclinics were for inferior doctors. This changed during 1965–67. There had to be an overall change since many worked at the polyclinics because they were required to and not because they wanted to."[53] Despite the new ideology proclaiming the importance of preventive medicine, doctors and other clinicians often continued to perceive health as the mere absence of disease.[54] A change in attitudes did occur, largely through the education of the next generation of practitioners.

Discord also arose regarding the role of health care professionals in determining policy. Doctors tend to be autonomous, confident that their own method is the best. What happens when their approach diverges from official policy, the community, or their colleagues? There was widespread disagreement, for example, over parents who wished to "live-in" with a hospitalized child. Dr. Felipe Cárdenas described a father who had to walk three hours every day to see his son, who was hospitalized with gastroenteritis in Guantánamo province.[55] Most doctors and nurses strongly opposed letting parents sleep in a child's hospital room, fearing that they would be a nuisance. But Dr. Enzo Dueñas recalled his experience at Lenin Hospital in Holguín during a shortage of nurses: "We had to have mothers taking care of their children. Now, the mother is with the child in the hospital and is not upset."[56] Cárdenas agreed that "the mother is the person who knows the child best, such as when he last used the bathroom or vomited. She needs to be involved in the care."[57] When the government decided to implement the policy of live-in parents, it proved very popular and resulted in shorter hospital stays for children. In general, the government sided with parents and the community during such disputes.

The effort to recruit more doctors continued through the decade. Women, whose career choices had traditionally been limited to teaching and nursing, now flooded into Cuban medical schools, making up 50 percent of students by 1970.[58] Government campaigns to boost medical school enrollment included personal appeals by Fidel, and by 1970 applications to medical school comprised 30 percent of all university applications.[59]

Nevertheless, the stress of medical school in Cuba during the 1960s was enough to cause almost half of students to drop out.[60] One program to retain students created *alumnos ayudantes* (student helpers, or peer tutors). Dr. María Luísa Lima, who now teaches at the Latin American School of Medicine, began medical school in 1965, when she was seventeen. She explained that the *ayudantes* were those who had done well in basic sciences and were closely tutored by doctors, so they could help others through those courses. The *ayudantes* both expanded the reach of professors and were themselves potential new faculty.[61]

Despite these efforts, the country still faced a shortage of doctors in 1969. As Peter Bourne and others have acknowledged: "The departure of thousands of doctors severely hurt the ability in the short term to provide health care for all, a major commitment of the regime."[62] But could their absence simultaneously have enhanced Cuba's ability to design its new medical system? I asked Cuban historian Hedelberto López how difficult it would have been to implement the changes of the 1960s, including the development of polyclinics, if the counterrevolutionary physicians had stayed. He replied, "Of course, the revolution in medicine would have been impossible if doctors had not fled the country. They would have disrupted everything."[63] Julia Sweig agrees that concerns over potential interference shaped revolutionary leaders' outlook: "Despite worries about losses of skilled professionals, Cuban authorities preferred that those who wanted no part of the revolution leave the island."[64] In effect, the departure of half of Cuba's doctors to Miami in the 1960s proved a double-edged sword: it cut into Cubans' health care, depriving millions of desperately needed health services, as the other edge cut off the ability of obstructionists to disrupt the building of a new medical world.

Navarro notes that, by the end of the decade, the number of graduating physicians was greater than the number who had left the country.[65] Although true, this overlooks Cuban population growth during the 1960s.[66] The issue is not merely the absolute number of doctors, but the ratio of doctors to patients.

Another factor complicating estimation of changes in the doctor-to-patient ratio during the first decade of the revolution is that Cuban researchers retabulated the number of physicians leaving the island. In 2015 Dr. Francisco Rojas Ochoa documented that the claim that half the physicians left was "a mistake that has been very frequently repeated."[67] Historical records from MINSAP showed that 2772 of the 6,286 Cuban doctors who practiced medicine in January 1959 left during 1959–68. This means that 44.1 percent departed, a number that is a bit less than half.

Table 2.1 combines figures from Rojas Ochoa for total number of doctors and the number who left from 1959 to 1968, Capote Mir's data for the number of medical students graduating annually, and information regarding Cuba's annual population.[68] It also projects

TABLE 2.1: Physicians and Population in Cuba, 1959–1976

Year	(A) Doctors	(B) Left Cuba	(C) Grad-uates	(D) Attrition Rate (%)	Population	Population Increase (%)	Doctors per 1,000 Cubans	Cubans per doctor
1959	6,286	42		2.00	6,901,000		0.91	1,098
1960	5,946	582	728	2.00	7,027,000	1.83	0.85	1,182
1961	5,472	778	335	2.00	7,134,000	1.52	0.77	1,304
1962	5,793	194	434	2.00	7,254,000	1.68	0.80	1,252
1963	6,239	161	334	2.00	7,415,000	2.22	0.84	1,188
1964	6,555	188	312	2.00	7,612,000	2.66	0.86	1,161
1965	6,815	214	395	2.00	7,810,000	2.60	0.87	1,146
1966	6,862	227	380	2.00	7,985,000	2.24	0.86	1,164
1967	6,960	197	433	2.00	8,139,000	1.93	0.86	1,169
1968	7,200	189	616	2.00	8,284,000	1.78	0.87	1,151
1969	7,474	196	940	2.00	8,421,000	1.65	0.89	1,127
1970	8,054	196	700	2.00	8,569,100	1.76	0.94	1,064
1971	8,387	196	535	2.00	8,692,000	1.43	0.96	1,036
1972	8,551	196	390	2.00	8,862,000	1.96	0.96	1,036
1973	8,571	196	1,047	2.00	9,036,000	1.96	0.95	1,054
1974	9,233	196	1,124	2.00	9,194,000	1.75	1.00	996
1975	9,958	196	1,361	2.00	9,299,000	1.14	1.07	934
1976	10,900	196	1,477	2.00	9,430,000	1.41	1.16	865

For the years 1959–1968, the number of doctors (A) and the number of doctors who left (B) is from Rojas Ochoa. For all years, the number of doctors who graduated is from Capote Mir. For the years 1969–1976, the number of doctors who left is estimated as 196 (average of doctors who left during 1963–1968) and the number of doctors in Cuba (A) is estimated as the number of doctors during the previous year minus the number of doctors who left (B) plus the number of doctors who graduated (C) minus a 2% attrition of doctors (from death, retirement, or change of profession).

SOURCE: Rojas Ochoa, "The Number of Physicians in Cuba, 1959–1968"; Navarro, "Health, Health Services, and Health Planning in Cuba"; Capote Mir, *La Evolución de los Servicios de Salud y la Estructura Socioeconómica en Cuba*; http://populstat.info.

the number departing Cuba during 1968–76 based on the average number of those who left during 1963–68 and an assumption of a 2 percent attrition rate of physicians (due to death, retirement or change of profession), which allows for an estimation of the number of physicians during 1969–76.

Including data for the annual rate of population increase in the table provides a much better calculation of when Cuba recovered from the loss of physicians. The 6,239 doctors in Cuba by 1963 almost matched the 6,286 at the beginning of 1959. But the population increase meant that the doctor-to-patient ratio was still below the 1959 level. The 1959 ratio of .91 physicians per 1,000 people was probably attained early in 1970. This suggests that recovery of the pre-revolutionary doctor-to-patient ratio was most likely reached a couple of years earlier than Danielson's estimate of 1972.[67]

Whichever date is used, Cuba's medical coordinators were expecting a future decrease in the need for doctors. By the early 1970s, they were both preparing a quota to reduce the medical acceptance rate to 20 percent of all university applicants and encouraging medical students to transfer into other programs.[68] This reflected the integration of divergent aspects of medicine as a system.

By the end of the revolution's first decade, the *policlínicos integrales* had taken a qualitative leap from expanding access to medical attention to conceiving and implementing a novel approach to health care as a whole. Through their practice, the clinics showed that it was possible to overcome the deficiencies of capitalist medicine and develop the collective consciousness required for a new system to take root.

Many lessons of the first decade of Cuban medicine had been anticipated before the revolution confirmed them. It became clear that health care could only be improved if a country simultaneously addressed necessities such as food, housing, and education; medical campaigns must be based on mass participation; obstructive institutions such as mutualism could be overcome by creating a better method of care delivery before abolishing the old one; an institution could be improved by undertaking two contradictory processes simultaneously (such as centralizing and decentralizing medicine); and, despite the short-term damage of almost three thousand doctors leaving, the long-term renovation of medicine was enhanced by their absence.

These lessons laid the foundations for the unique Cuban network of clinics. Defined geographic areas offered single points of patient entry into a system that combined preventive care with treatment. Through decentralized control of their own functions, the Cuban clinics quickly gained an equal footing with hospitals.

Still, as the 1970s began, many unanswered questions remained. Could reallocation of resources continue to improve health even as Cuba remained poor and blockaded? Would the system of *policlínicos integrales* be able to reduce infant mortality? With the ratio of doctors to population approaching pre-1959 levels, would fewer students be admitted to medical school, or would unforeseen circumstances require a continued expansion of enrollment? Would *policlínicos integrales* continue as they existed during the period 1964 to 1969, or would other structures and services replace or alter them?

— 3 —

CUBA'S FIRST MILITARY DOCTORS

Cuba's deployment of military doctors to Africa in the 1960s was a secret, known only at the highest level of government. In fact, accounts of these hidden efforts were not published until the beginning of the twenty-first century. Many forces during that decade pulled Cuba toward struggles in sub-Saharan Africa. First was the mushrooming of popular movements across the globe. The U.S. civil rights movement was joined by millions opposing the war in Vietnam. Zaire won independence from Belgium in June 1960, and the popular Patrice Lumumba became its first prime minister. After leading the National Liberation Front to victory over French domination in 1962, Ahmed Ben Bella was elected as the first president of Algeria. In August 1966, Mao Zedong launched the Great Proletarian Cultural Revolution to thwart the growth of capitalism in China. May 1968 saw a huge left upsurge in France that went beyond the Communist Party.

The second force pushing Cuba's foreign policy was U.S. imperialism. Two decades earlier, the United States experimented with nuclear extermination in Hiroshima and Nagasaki. In the previous decade, the United States had slaughtered roughly 20 percent of the population of North Korea and the Central Intelligence Agency (CIA) engineered the overthrow of the progressive Jacobo Arbenz government in Guatemala. Fresh on the mind of Cubans was the connivance of John and Bobby Kennedy in the 1961 Bay of Pigs invasion and the 1962 missile crisis. At around the same time as the CIA was strategizing about how to poison Lumumba, it was also launching its efforts to kill Fidel Castro.[1] Asserting dominion over Latin America, Lyndon Johnson invaded the Dominican Republic in 1965.

In the meantime, the Soviet Union was not acting like a reliable ally. The USSR had not sent troops to fight in Korea and did not do so in Vietnam, even after the massive U.S. buildup following the 1964 Gulf of Tonkin incident. Nikita Khrushchev had settled the missile crisis without bothering to consult Fidel, and Khrushchev's successor, Leonid Brezhnev, made clear that Cuba should accept the subordinate status of being a sugar producer for the Soviet bloc.

Furthermore, Latin American communist parties did not take kindly to Cuba's "foco theory" of revolution. Those parties centered on urban working-class movements while the Cuban leadership looked to a dedicated vanguard in the countryside, garnering support through armed struggle. As Che Guevara explained, "A small group of men who are determined, supported by the people, and not afraid of death . . . can overcome a regular army. This was the lesson of the Cuban Revolution."[2] Unlike countries in Latin America, those in Africa did not have established communist parties hostile to guerrilla efforts.[3] With at least a third of Cubans being of African heritage, Cuban leaders felt beckoned from across the Atlantic.

Hope Meets Reality in Africa

Despite efforts by the United States to isolate Cuba, by 1964 the island had embassies in the African countries of Algeria, Egypt, Ghana, Guinea, Mali, Morocco, and Tanzania. In January 1961, Lumumba was murdered by allies of Moise Tshombe, and in 1964 followers of Lumumba, the Simbas (lions), began a guerrilla struggle that had strong revolutionary potential and routed government forces.[4]

In December 1964, Che began a three-month trek through Algeria, Ghana, the Congo, Guinea, Mali, Benin, Tanzania, and Egypt. Planning to lead an African revolutionary project himself, Che went to develop strategies and agreements with liberation movements. During his January 1965 meeting with leaders in Tanzania, Che emphasized the lessons from the Simba rebellion and proposed Zaire as the location for centralized training. African leaders disagreed with him, each wanting training camps in their own country.[5]

The more Che came to know the heads of several organizations, the more skeptical he became. He observed that they "live comfortably in hotels and have turned rebellion into a profession, at times lucrative."[6] Once on the battlefield, his doubts were confirmed:

> Che had been told that he would find several thousand well-armed Simbas, eager to fight. There were, in fact, some 1,000 to 1,500 widely dispersed rebels who had no idea how to maintain their modern weapons. . . . They lacked a unified command.
>
> The scouting teams . . . brought back grim reports from the fronts: idle rebels who . . . did not know how to use their firearms and showed no inclination to attack or to prepare to defend themselves. Everywhere chaos, disorganization, and lack of discipline.[7]

Cuban leaders, soldiers, and doctors wrote of their frustrations in Zaire. In November 1965, after a governmental coup, a Simba leader notified Che that they wanted to end the war. Che returned to Cuba with part of the unit he commanded, while others went to different African locations.[8]

The neighboring Congo's president was Alphonse Massamba-Débat, whose socialist views were similar to those of the Chinese Communist Party.[9] In August 1965, Fidel dispatched a unit to the Congo that joined the fifty or so Cubans already there. The group was headed by Jorge Risquet, who was the "descendant of an African slave, her white master, a Chinese indentured servant, and a Spanish immigrant."[10]

In the Congo, the Cubans discovered that the rhetoric of the country's leaders did not match their politics, which were fueled by opportunism and personal feuds. Since Fidel had charged Risquet with defending the Congo, when an attempted coup broke out on June 27, 1966, the Cubans came to the defense of the government. Wanting to resolve the dispute diplomatically rather than by force, Risquet appointed a doctor to lead the maneuvers. The rebels backed down when confronted by the determination of the smaller number of Cubans. On July 6, the revolt ended with only one Congolese death.[11] It soon became clear to the Cubans that their major task in the Congo was protecting one faction from another. Risquet persuaded the Cuban government that the best thing for them to do was leave, which they soon did. Two years later, a successful coup overthrew Massamba-Débat's government.[12]

The uprising against the Portuguese in Guinea-Bissau stood in sharp contrast to the Congolese and Zairean movements. Even U.S. intelligence reports described Guinea-Bissau as having "Africa's most successful liberation movement."[13] During his 1965 journey through Africa, Che spoke with the Bissau-Guinean and Cape Verdean Amílcar Cabral, head of the African Party for the Independence of Guinea and Cape Verde (PAIGC, the acronym in Portuguese).[14]

Fidel recognized the importance of the Non-Aligned Movement, which brought together third world countries breaking from the yoke of imperialism. He persuaded those organizing the Tricontinental Congress to meet in Havana on January 3, 1966, and invited Latin American groups dedicated to armed struggle. It was there that Fidel and Cabral first met and spoke extensively. Fidel promised Cabral doctors, military instructors, and mechanics.[15] Both made impressive speeches to the Congress's delegates, and Fidel emerged as a champion of revolutionary movements.

For a critical year, Victor Dreke headed Cuba's military undertaking in Guinea-Bissau. Dreke was a black commander who received extremely high praise from Che for his efforts in Zaire. Dreke was impressed by the discipline of the PAIGC, and by the time he returned to Cuba in late 1968, Cabral's forces had strengthened their position. The Portuguese lost ground even while increasing their troops from 20,000 to 25,000.[16] Cuba never had more than sixty soldiers in

Guinea-Bissau, which was one of the ways Cabral kept the PAIGC under his command. The other way was restricting foreign military aid only to Cubans. Yet the Cubans' roles as military advisers and teachers proved invaluable. When Fidel went to Africa in 1972, the PAIGC was the only force on the continent successfully fighting against a white regime.[17]

In this period, Cuba also played minor roles in Angola, Cameroon, Equatorial Guinea, Tanzania, and possibly other countries.[18] Here, however, we will focus on Zaire, the Congo, and Guinea-Bissau, which were, by far, its major arenas. Much of the information regarding the experiences of Cuban physicians in Africa is from extensive interviews with military doctors deployed in the three countries, as well as Tanzania.

WHITE DOCTORS, BLACK SOLDIERS

Cuban doctors going to Africa were almost all white, whereas its troops were almost all black. Before the revolution, it was very rare for black people to become doctors, although they rose quickly to high positions in the revolutionary military. Race was critical in every aspect of the African conflicts.

The United States had strong advantages over Cuba in its influence in Africa: it could offer vastly more economic aid and wield the political power of its European allies, accrued by their history of conquest and ongoing domination. But throughout the 1960s, the United States was increasingly tied up in Vietnam, and its ongoing racism repulsed people around the globe. Racism in the white regimes of Africa was also blatant and horrific. The *Observer* reported that mercenaries paid to put down the Simba rebellion "not only shoot and hang prisoners after torturing them, but use them for target practice and gamble over the number of shots to kill them." One mercenary wrote of the "White Giants" in his memoirs: "Tall, vigorous Boers from South Africa; long-legged, slim and muscular Englishmen from Rhodesia—who would restore, in Zaire, the white man to his proper place."[19]

African resistance leaders realized that they could use to their advantage the inability of racists to tell one group of black people from another. The revolutionaries in Zaire requested that the Cubans sent to aid them be black so they could pass undetected by U.S. and European spies. Cabral asked Cuban officials to send technicians who were "black or dark mulattoes so that they would blend in with his people," a request that fell into place with the PAIGC's policy of denying that their actions involved any foreigners.[20]

When Fidel asked Dreke to select troops who would serve in Zaire with Che, he specified that he had to "choose a platoon of men who have shown their mettle, who are all volunteers and who are dark-skinned blacks." Neither Dr. Rodrigo Álvarez Cambras nor Dr. Julián Álvarez Blanco knew that Africa was their destination until they saw that almost all the combatants in the training camps were black.[21]

This led to very different experiences for those traveling by ship to Africa. Dr. Álvarez Cambras remembers episodes of Pavlovian conditioning when traveling aboard the Soviet ship *Félix Dzerzhinsky*:

> Since the doctors were all white, there were no problems with anyone seeing us. But the troops were all black, and, in order to make sure that none of the passengers or U.S. spy planes would guess the purpose of the mission, they had to stay in the lower deck of the ship, which was hot and had poor ventilation. Occasionally, they could come out briefly at night.
>
> Since the Russian food was very strong with disagreeable odors, the comrades who had to stay below without fresh air would get nauseous and vomit when they smelled it. The captain had a gong that he hit in front of a microphone to announce that it was time to eat. Some of the comrades started vomiting when they heard the gong.
>
> At that point, I told Risquet that he had to tell the ship's captain to stop banging the gong. He replied that it was I, as a doctor, who had to have that conversation with the captain. When I did, that robust Russian failed to understand the situation and argued that it was a tradition that he could not violate.[22]

Though the white doctors could lean over the side of the ship to vomit, it must have been profoundly unpleasant for the black troops confined to the lower deck. In response, and to the outrage of the Russian captain, the Cubans stole the gong and heaved it into the Atlantic![23]

The strategy of recruiting black troops significantly slowed the ability of Western powers to detect Cuban involvement. A British adviser in Zaire observed that U.S. agents looked "for whites and their eyes . . . passed over Cuban blacks or mulattoes." The same was true for the Congo, where bewildered officials from the United States, France, West Germany, and England "were unable to ascertain how many Cubans were in the Congo." A Belgian ambassador could not tell if there were one hundred or eight hundred Cubans since "they are difficult to pick out because they are all colored."[24] It was likely a serious affront to the dignity of white supremacists to see black Cubans so successfully bamboozling them.

Recruiting Doctors

Western observers could only be successfully deceived about Cuban involvement if Cuba's own recruits were not informed about their destination. Rodolfo Puente was the only one of nine physicians interviewed by Hedelberto López Blanch who was openly told where he was going (in his case, the Congo).[25] Others were led to believe that they were going to Algeria, Vietnam, or "other lands" or instructed to tell their families that they would be studying in the Soviet Union.[26]

The physicians were accustomed to disruption in their careers. Of the nine interviewed by López Blanch, two had to delay beginning medical school because Fulgencio Batista closed it at the end of 1956. The other seven started school before the 1956 closing, but had to halt their studies and resume them after the 1959 revolution.

Waiting to discover where exactly they would serve was just one indication of the vital importance of their mission. Additionally, every one of the nine physicians interviewed in *Historias Secretas* met some combination of Fidel, Raúl Castro, Che, MINSAP (the Cuban Health

Department) head José Ramón Machado, Commander Risquet, Commander Dreke, and Cabral before, during, and/or after their trip to Africa. Preparing to leave for Zaire, Rafaél Zerquera recalled that "April 10, 1965, was the happiest day of my life because I was interviewed by Fidel Castro."[27] Shortly after arriving in Zaire, Diego Lagomasino "gave Che a suitcase with asthma medicine and bullets for an M1 gun. Meeting someone like Che had a big impact."[28] Héctor Vera spoke with Fidel upon returning from Zaire: "Fidel asked about sicknesses, malaria, how we were able to diagnose, and what treatments we used. After chatting, he told us that we could not divulge anything about the mission."[29]

Before departing for the Congo, Álvarez Cambras describes having breakfast with Fidel:

He spoke to us of Africa in general without specifying the country. He asked if we had pistols, and I said, yes, a P38. He told his assistant to find a better weapon and he brought a Stich of twenty shots. Fidel saw that I wasn't wearing a watch and told me that it was important for a doctor going to war to have one. He took off one of the two watches he was wearing, a Longines, and gave it to me.[30]

When Diego Lagomasino did his postgraduate Rural Medical Service (RMS) in Santo Tomás, he worked alone and "had to be the doctor, nurse, distribute medications, and look for supplies."[31] This multitasking helped prepare him for Africa. Zerquera explains that when he graduated his RMS was used as a screening to see if he was suitable for the Zaire mission:

A document circulated asking where we would like to do our RMS and I wrote "wherever the revolution needs me." José Ramón Machado of MINSAP called me to his office and said that there was a conflict zone in the Sierra Maestra, where a group had burned the medical post and killed the doctor. He asked me if I was still willing to go.[32]

Zerquera replied that he would go where Machado assigned him. After a short stint in the Sierra Maestra, Machado called him back to let him know that an important but highly risky international mission awaited him and Zerquera was soon on his way to Zaire.

Once they learned of their destinations, the doctors still had little idea of what was in store for them. Luís Peraza recalled that all he "knew about Africa was the Tarzan movies." Impressions of their experiences differed sharply according to country, with Zaire being the gloomiest. Toward the end of the period of Cuban military support in Zaire, Che called a meeting of Communist Party members and asked who still thought that they could win. Only two military leaders and two doctors raised their hands, and Che concluded that they might have been showing him personal support. Che then asked who would be willing to fight until death and all the hands went up.[33]

Zerquera remembered how the Simbas in Zaire did not seem interested in preparing for a guerrilla struggle: "It was an experience, but it wasn't pleasant. If it had been a sacrifice with a reward, I would have felt satisfied. But it was not rewarding."[34]

The Congo inspired different feelings in Justo Piñeiro. "The population identified with us," he explained. "We bought things from them. We went to the same places and knew the local people from seeing them on the street."[35]

By far, however, the most positive memories were of Guinea-Bissau. Domingo Díaz knew "many brave Guinean officers and soldiers who would have given their lives to prevent a Cuban from falling into the hands of the enemy."[36] Dr. Milton Hechevarría emphasized that when he got back to Cuba, he couldn't forget Guinea-Bissau.[37]

Whatever country they went to, Cuban doctors faced a combination of stressful conditions that they were unlikely to have experienced at home: incredibly rough terrain, enemy fire, and unpleasant, dangerous animals. Diego Lagomasino recalled facing serious physical challenges when his group arrived in Zaire:

We had to go to the base camp that was on the top of a high ridge. We left at six in the morning and at seven in the evening were still climbing. Never in my life had I seen a ridge that tall. I thought I was going to die.[38]

Looking back on the same walk, Héctor Vera felt like he could not bear the weight of his pistol, ammunition, medical supplies, and personal belongings in his knapsack. He was saved by a Zairean boy who motioned that he would carry it for him.[39]

In Guinea-Bissau, Díaz went on strenuous walks for seven or eight days, on roads with deep holes that could not be seen after it rained. "In this region, we didn't measure time with a watch," Díaz recounted. Instead, time was measured by "distance, which is to say one day's walk, half a day's walk." He concluded that the terrain was so rough that "in Cuba there was no possibility of training for this type of event."[40]

In addition to the challenges of the terrain, there were military dangers. To avoid detection by the enemy, Héctor Vera's group crossed Lake Tanganyika with several Simbas who began lighting matches to see where they were going. The Cubans in the boat told them not to because there was a gasoline motor that could catch on fire. However, there was no other way to see and they continued with the matches. Upon arriving in Zaire, they had not traveled fifty meters before they had to fall to the ground as enemy planes flew overhead.[41]

In Guinea-Bissau, the Portuguese attacked Amado Alfonso Delgado's group with napalm, while fifteen helicopters landed to hunt them. They survived by running from seven in the morning until five in the afternoon.[42]

The doctors encountered insects, reptiles, and other creatures they had never seen before. In an emergency military undertaking in the Congo, Álvarez Cambras saw anthills so tall that they prevented their plane from landing.[43] Fleeing from the Portuguese in Guinea-Bissau, Delgado recalls bumping into an enormous beehive:

I had over three hundred stings. Only ten were dangerous and can send a person into shock. But I was under so much tension that my body was producing steroids, which is exactly the treatment used. None of the stings became inflamed and the other six with me had the same luck.[44]

While none of Cuba's snakes are poisonous, many *are* in the Congo where Julián Álvarez thought he ran across them everywhere.[45]

Waters in Guinea-Bissau were often inhospitable. Díaz described walking through a lake for hours with water up to their chests. "It was full of leeches and they advised me to tie my pants tight and walk with my arms up so they could not get in. When we got out we were attacked by mosquitoes that bit through my coat." One day, Díaz and his comrades found that

> the Corubal and Gaba Rivers met where they emptied into the sea. It was like an arm of the sea where there were sharks, hippopotamuses, and crocodiles. As we crossed in canoes made from tree trunks, they told me to be careful because a man had recently fallen in and never reappeared.[46]

Military Doctors at Work

Physicians found working conditions to be quite different from those in Cuban polyclinics. It was very clear to Virgilio Camacho that although he was a doctor, he was armed because at any moment he might have to participate in combat.[47] The Cuban doctors practiced in small groups. In the Congo, the group Álvarez Cambras was part of included a surgeon, an orthopedist, and two pediatricians. Later, they were joined by an anesthesiologist nurse and dentists.[48] In 1966, Díaz traveled toward Guinea-Bissau as one of nine physicians. Once there, he was assigned to Saará in the northern region where they were "the only three doctors and there were no Cuban nurses." They worked closely with several young Guineans and trained them as nurses.[49]

Since the Cuban staff rotated and PAIGC policy was to understate the extent of their involvement, some historians are not aware of the more than forty Cuban doctors who served in Guinea-Bissau between 1966 and 1974, as writer Piero Gleijeses carefully documents.[50]

The physicians were forced to minimize their use of modest resources. When Delgado reached his assigned eastern front in Guinea-Bissau, he found that the hospital grounds consisted of "four huts: one for the wounded; one a kitchen; one for supplies; and one, a little farther away, for the doctor."[51]

Another low-profile and low-resource mission was the one in Tanzania. Juan Antonio Sánchez participated in the military mission there from 1969 to 1970 as a "medical internist at Pemba Island. Cuba had permission from the Tanzanian government as long as their presence was secret. There were no Cuban troops, only three doctors." Their "operating room had been a garage."[52]

The priority for Cuban doctors was always the health of combatants. They were treated for bullet wounds, fractures, and health issues such as hernias and tropical diseases. There were many surgeries, including one in which Héctor Vera participated. "Four men who had been injured by a grenade arrived," Vera recounts. "The one who was seriously injured was operated on at night and survived. We put him on a table; Che held a lantern; Oliva gave him anesthesia; Tabito operated; Lagomasino worked as an assistant; and I observed."[53]

Camacho served in the southern front of Guinea-Bissau where the Portuguese frequently ambushed civilians who helped supply the military. Several Cubans died or were injured in these attacks.[54] Delgado describes the difficulties of surgery during combat:

We operated whenever there were battles. Small reconnaissance planes passed overhead frequently, and, when they returned multiple times, we moved the camp because an attack was almost certain to follow. The hospital was burned four times. Every time a plane flew overhead twice, they attacked us. . . . We were between two rivers. Planes and boats kept coming by and destroyed almost all the canoes we could use to flee. . . . Most of the time we operated in places where we could set up a tiny hospital. They brought us people who had stepped on a mine or were wounded in an ambush. Almost always, the wounded arrived at night and we had to operate by

the light of bundles of grass. I did about fifty operations like
this, including several amputations. We cut dry grass, folded it
over, tied it with straw, and used it as a candle. Sometimes we
couldn't see what we were operating on, even with eight or ten
wicks like this.[55]

Other than Military Medicine

Cubans felt obligated to treat civilians injured in attacks, which meant
that there was an overlap between military and non-military medicine. Delgado became acutely aware that a lack of specialists had its
costs. He describes one experience in Guinea-Bissau:

A bomb fell very close to a woman and injured her abdomen. Since
I didn't have my assistant with me, I had to read from a booklet to
find out how to apply anesthesia. I had to open her abdomen to
see if she had peritonitis. I gave her local anesthesia, and just as I
was about to give her general anesthesia, a plane dropped a bomb
very close to us. The woman jumped up with her wound half open
and ran away. I never saw her again. Later I learned that she had
been found dead four kilometers from the tiny hospital.[56]

Díaz had a more positive experience in the northern front:

One day in Saará, they brought us a boy about four years old
named Kumba, who had a large wound in his left leg. His good
spirit impressed us; he didn't shed a tear or show pain. A few
hours before, the Portuguese attacked a nearby village that had
no combatants and no protection. Luckily, they were able to
bring this little boy to our small rural hospital. We cleaned the
very dirty wound and partially sutured it because we didn't want
future complications, such as gangrene. During all the treatment
without anesthesia, Kumba continued as before, without a tear
or expression of pain.[57]

Cuban officials knew that the behavior of doctors toward civilians was as important for diplomatic relationships as troop discipline was for military advances. When Cuban physicians first went to Algeria in 1963, Raúl Castro issued a strict code of conduct that included a prohibition of alcohol and intimate relations with women, and demanded absolute respect for Algerian traditions. Che spoke to physicians in Zaire of the moral aspect of their mission: "I don't want any scandal. Anyone who is undisciplined will have to be counseled or sent back to Cuba." A couple of years later, the Cuban command in Guinea-Bissau replaced a doctor accused of not showing respect for local customs.[58]

The importance of this respect grew as Cubans and Africans became closer. Unlike Catholic and Protestant missionary doctors, who stayed at fixed locations and required Africans to come to them, Cubans went on long walks to isolated villages to provide care. As Zaireans learned of the arrival of Cuban doctors, "peasants from the surrounding area flocked in." Before the Cubans arrived, only nine doctors had provided care for almost a million Congolese. Hugo Spadafora, a Panamanian who was the only foreign doctor with the PAIGC, wrote that when the Cuban physicians arrived with medicine and equipment "the quality of the hospital's care increased exponentially."[59]

The guidelines laid out by Raúl and Che served Cuban efforts well. While their military allies in Zaire were often accused of mistreating local people, there were "no reports of the Cubans perpetrating any crimes or acts of violence against the population."[60]

Instead, the Cubans won people's trust by doing countless simple procedures. These included tooth extractions, operations for hernias and cataracts, and treatments for high fever, diarrhea, confusion, stomachaches, and shoulder pain. In Tanzania, Piñeiro recalled that "most patients were civilian and a few were military. The most frequent problems were malnutrition, malaria, pneumonia, and parasites."[61]

Delgado learned to treat parasitic diseases he had never seen in Cuba:

I saw whole villages with trachoma, an infection of the eyes and eyelids that leaves people blind. I visited villages where almost everyone was blind. I saw people with advanced leprosy, without fingers. There was a sickness, *miasis*, produced by a fly bite that causes an abscess from which worms grow. Another produces boils on the body, called onchocerciasis, which is a type of filaria. This disease has a special treatment. There is a worm that gets under the skin and the Guineans use a little stick to which they fasten a palm thread and put it in the boil and roll it around until they pull out an enormous worm called "the worm of Guinea." There are many parasites and harmful insects, such as the jigger flea (*nigua*), which gets under people's skin in dry weather and causes boils. You have to extract the parasite, which looks like a tick.[62]

Perhaps one of the most unexpected tragedies was a Cuban soldier dying from eating a strawberry. He had a perforated ulcer and no idea how acidic the fruit could be. "By the time he reached me," Díaz remembers, "he was in agony. We did all we could to stop the bleeding, and since we didn't have surgical instruments, we tried to move him to the small hospital in Boké. But he died on the road."[63]

Though the Cubans tried to attend to civilian medical needs, operations had to be authorized by the PAIGC area director due to shortage of materials. This required creative searches for alternative materials, such as using coconut water (which is sterile) in intravenous fluids. On multiple occasions, Camacho "had to suture patients with domestic sewing thread," which led to deal-making with local thread vendors.[64]

Truly International Medicine

The riches of Africa were being drained as its peoples lay crippled or dying from curable diseases, which did not pique the interest of wealthy Western investors. This was the case with polio. Álvarez Cambras gives a picture of what he witnessed when he arrived in the Congo:

Many suffered from polio. I visited an asylum attended by a single nun that was full of children with the disease. The children were crawling across the floor in very bare surroundings. The nun didn't have supplies or staff to deal with them. I operated on dozens of these children. . . . The French had left nothing of the infrastructure; there were no lawyers or engineers, and only two native doctors.[65]

Dr. Puente was the manager and one of the principal advocates for a polio vaccination campaign. He ran into two Soviet medical staff who were vaccinating as one of their duties. He asked for five thousand doses, which they happily gave him, and made arrangements with the mayor to vaccinate students. Realizing the seriousness of the situation and knowing that Cuba had recently conducted its own polio vaccination campaign, Puente called MINSAP in Havana for permission to take on a similar endeavor. MINSAP director Machado approved and assigned Dr. Helenio Ferrer, Cuba's Director of Epidemiology, to fly to Moscow for the vaccines. The Soviets agreed to provide 200,000 doses to the Congo for about four thousand pesos. Following appeals by the Cubans, they agreed to donate the vaccines, which arrived in June 1966.[66]

There were not enough doctors and nurses to administer the vaccines, but since they were placed in caramel candies, it was possible to train others to distribute them. In cooperation with the Congolese government, its militia, the Federation of Women, and Cuban troops, Ferrer coordinated the vaccination of over 61,000 children in the first such campaign in Africa.[67]

Unfortunately, the attempted coup of June 27, 1966, blocked administration of the second dose. Accounts tend to be vague about whether blocking the second dose prevented the first dose from being effective. However, when asked, Piñeiro, who was in the Congo from September 1966 to November 1967, explained, "As a result of not getting the second dose, there would be the same rate of polio." He returned to the Congo in May 1969 and witnessed the Congolese Ministry of Public Health administering both doses, which were provided by the Soviets. He strongly believed that the earlier joint experience with the Cubans was critical in making the 1969 effort successful.[68]

In Guinea-Bissau, Díaz's group found themselves with no Cuban nurses, so they trained several local youth. They were so impressed with the work of the Guineans that they sought and obtained permission from Cabral to bring four back to attend Cuban nursing school, from which they later graduated.[69]

This was not the only time that Cuba extended its educational resources to Africans. A few years earlier in the Congo, Cuban doctors noticed dedicated young people studying at night under streetlights. They asked the Congolese government about sending some of them to Cuba to study. The Congolese government agreed and, on January 24, 1966, 254 youths boarded a ship for Havana. This was the first time a significant number of foreign scholarship students went to Cuba. Nevertheless, there were problems. Rather than choosing students strictly on the basis of academic performance, many were selected according to personal connections or bribes. By late 1967, more than one hundred had returned home, per their own or the Cuban government's request. Despite this, by 1978, twenty-five had Cuban medical degrees and others graduated as lab technicians or engineers.[70]

Cuban authorities soon decided that its military forces would leave Africa. Yet medical personnel would continue with replacement teams of "pediatricians, orthopedics, surgeons, and ear-nose-throat specialists who would be civilian rather than military doctors."[71]

PHYSICIANS, HEAL EACH OTHER

Cuban doctors provided preventive care and treatment not only to troops and civilians, but also to themselves. The most famous example was Che. With him in Zaire, Zerquera remembered the day Che's malaria was complicated by an asthma attack. Zerquera worried about the possibility of having to tell Fidel that he let Che die there. Che was not an exception. Delgado, for example, treated himself three times for malaria.[72]

Camacho spoke about how, soon after his arrival, acute jaundice caused another doctor, Jesús Pérez, to return to Cuba, leaving him with only one other doctor at their medical post. A year later, he was transferred to head the military hospital in Guinea-Bissau's southern front because a doctor there was ill.[73]

The long walks and physical exhaustion of battlefield medicine took their toll. When Díaz arrived in Guinea-Bissau, he weighed 180 pounds. He left twenty months later, weighing only a hundred pounds. He had also experienced the unusual danger of disappearing shoes:

> I returned to the base after it was completely destroyed, and I could not find any of my belongings, not even my tennis shoes. This type of footwear was the best for the circumstances, since we had to cross many rivers, and they dried much more quickly than boots and were a lot lighter. . . . During the first long walks, I lost all of my toenails . . . my feet were constantly wet and the hiking was constant . . . and in Cuba I had the habit of walking five kilometers every day.[74]

Some of the most unpleasant surprises awaited doctors upon completing their African assignments. Delgado recounted:

> The year that we returned, almost all of us tested positive for filaria in our blood. In the subtype loiasis, it goes from the vital organs to the eyes, leaving the person blind. This was precisely the type we had. Reading about it scared me because, at the time, it was said that there was no guaranteed cure. We were treated in a hospital for two months.[75]

Camacho was also more than a little nervous:

> I had filaria, which doesn't exist in Cuba, and I had no idea until I passed through the checkpoint. It required a double treatment, both for the adult parasite and the larva. They didn't have the medicine in Conakry and had to look elsewhere. Finally, I

received the intravenous injections and took pills. . . . We arrived in Cuba in January 1968.[76]

IMPACT, REFLECTION, UNANSWERED QUESTIONS

By the end of the 1960s, when the Cuban revolutionary government had been in power for only ten years, doctors had been through four different situations in Africa: (1) in Algeria, they had treated only civilians; (2) in Zaire, the rebels had shown little enthusiasm for victory; (3) in the Congo, the government's commitment had proven to be empty rhetoric; but (4) in Guinea-Bissau, there had been a successful military uprising with a strong commander and dedicated troops.

Cuba knew that the United States could invade at any time. As a result of African expeditions and experience gained by military doctors, a new generation of physicians would be trained by those who had been through war and could teach others how to treat combat victims. Perhaps the most lamentable irony of Cuba's forays into Africa was that the country's most capable leader, Che, led guerrillas into Zaire, the least promising front. Since no Cuban leader had been to sub-Saharan Africa for more than one day, the strategy of going to Zaire was based on misinformation, solidarity with Cuba's own black population, and the defense of its revolution. When Che embarked on his last mission in Bolivia the following year, it was because he and Fidel agreed that Latin America must again occupy the foreground of Cuba's participation in armed struggles.[77]

The connection between the approach to medicine practiced on the island and the methods learned by its doctors overseas was limited.[78] Lessons from the experiences of the polio campaign in Cuba were adopted in the campaign in the Congo. Conversely, the exposure to medical issues in Africa was invaluable for developing Cuban understanding of tropical and infectious diseases. Nevertheless, nothing like Cuban polyclinics appeared in the battle conditions of Africa, where the necessity to provide emergency care was all-encompassing.

Still, Cuban engagement in Africa left a profound impact, both on the host countries and on the Cubans who went. Cuba learned that if students were to travel to the island for education, they must be screened for academic potential. The Congo became prepared to complete its own vaccination campaign. Guinea-Bissau recognized its debt to Cubans for its successful struggle for independence. "Many of our comrades are alive today only because of the Cuban medical assistance," noted PAIGC official Francisco Pereira. "The Cuban doctors really performed a miracle. I am eternally grateful to them: not only did they save lives, but they put their own lives at risk. They were truly selfless."[79]

White doctors who experienced the stressful conditions and parasitic diseases of Africa witnessed even greater sacrifices by black troops. One of the reasons that so many volunteered to serve in Africa was a feeling of urgency to spread the revolution. Later, Olvaldo Cárdenas spoke to Piero Gleijeses about this sense of urgency:

> We believed that at any moment [the United States was] going to strike us . . . and for us it was better to wage war abroad than in our own country. This was the strategy of "Two or Three Vietnams"; that is, distracting and dividing the enemy's forces. I never imagined then that I would be sitting [in a living room in Havana] talking about it now—we all assumed that we were going to die young.[80]

When the volunteers returned to Cuba, they did not march in parades or receive any type of public praise. There were no medals, celebrations, or material rewards. Bound to secrecy, decades passed before they could share their stories.[81] Yet the insights obtained by what they endured were essential for designing Cuban strategy, which is why Fidel grilled so many when they quietly arrived home.

Before 1959, dedication to revolutionary medicine was expressed by students and doctors demanding full treatment for Cubans in poor urban and rural areas. This became the foundation for doctors volunteering for international missions during the 1960s. With the dawn of the 1970s, the question remained: Would sacrifices by the first doctors going to Africa lead to medical staff playing a key role in toppling a major racist government on that continent?

— 4 —

FROM *POLICLÍNICOS COMUNITARIOS* TO FAMILY MEDICINE

The 1970s promised to be a difficult time for Cuba. Che Guevara, one of the one of the most inspiring leaders of the revolution, had been killed in October 1967. Furthermore, the decade began with the rabidly anti-communist Richard Nixon in the White House and with Cuba having somewhat chilly relations with both Moscow and Beijing. Finally, though Fidel Castro had hoped that the island would diversify its economy, Leonid Brezhnev made it clear that Cuba would continue to be a sugar monoproducer for the Eastern Bloc. Resigned to this fate, the revolutionary government announced that 1970 would be the year of the greatest sugar harvest in history. It set the production goal at ten million tons, which was almost double the 1968 harvest. Yet real production fell short of expectations, and workers taking time off from their jobs to work in the cane fields seriously damaged the economy. As a result, Cubans throughout the country participated in an intense discussion of the revolutionary process.

Since redesign of the medical system occurred at the same time, I asked Dr. Julio López Benítez if that transformation had been part of the broad process of self-examination . He responded negatively:

The failure of the sugar harvest and the change in polyclinics were completely different. We never sacrificed health care for other things. It was a moral mission. It was not compulsory for anyone to cut sugarcane. Doctors were not good at cutting cane, so, the ones who did it went back to practicing medicine to free others to cut cane.[1]

Yet even if the reorganization of medical clinics had little to do with Cuba's self-critique in response to the sugar harvest failure, the changes in the health system were highly significant ones. López recalls:

The change was patients going to clinics versus clinics going to the patient. The *policlínico integral* was a clinic of specialties, but they did not visit the community. The *policlínico comunitario* was based on visiting people in their communities.

FROM *POLICLÍNICOS INTEGRALES* TO *POLICLÍNICOS COMUNITARIOS*

Policlínicos integrales had begun in 1964, when Cuban medicine became strong enough to move beyond responding to the inadequacies of pre-revolutionary medicine and initiate a redesign of the system. Now, as medical planners became aware of problems with the first clinics, they laid the groundwork for the new *policlínicos comunitarios*. Though 1974 is given as the official date of the transformation, ideas for the new approach had appeared as early as 1969 and had existed in germinal form from the earliest days of medical revolution.[2]

The original *policlínicos integrales* had made tremendous accomplishments. They pulled a disparate array of care providers together. For the first time, there was a single point of entry into a health system, that kept coherent records for every patient. They incorporated millions of Cubans into the health system who had never even seen a doctor before. They also developed a nationwide system of preventive and curative care while providing a systematic approach to confronting a range of diseases.

Nevertheless, problems with *policlínicos integrales* emerged within five years of their creation. All basic care had fallen on their shoulders. Their duties had expanded so rapidly and become so complex that they found it difficult to provide all the services they were assigned.[3] Adding to the complexity was the continued separation of specialists. Physicians rarely worked together as a team. This meant that patients were passed from one specialist to another, not knowing who they would see during a follow-up visit.

The shuffling of patients between specialists was exacerbated in urban clinics where polyclinics were heavily staffed by residents on rotation.[4] The residents and their teachers tended to work separately from other physicians in the community. This resulted not only in patient dissatisfaction, but it also demoralized physicians who would hurry to refer patients to another specialist. Not having a patient followed by a single physician hindered the full integration of polyclinics into the community.

The frustrations that both patients and doctors experienced reflected structural contradictions between the goals of revolutionary health care and the way medicine was actually being practiced. An assessment conducted by the Ministry of Public Health (MINSAP) in the early 1970s identified a number of problems, concluding most physicians had not been trained as basic caregivers and had focused only on their specialties; doctors still believed the best care came from prestigious specialists; medicine continued to focus on curing disease while preventive health care received inadequate attention; specialists and hospitals always looked for more expensive technology, which threatened funding for clinics; and opportunities for community involvement in health care were lacking.[5]

For these reasons, doctors, patients, and the government were all ready for a big shakeup of the polyclinics. Some even asked if the polyclinics should continue to be so autonomous or if they should be placed under hospital supervision. Should the independent structure of the polyclinics be discarded?[6] The outcome of this self-examination of health delivery was a thoroughgoing redesign of clinics, which became known as "medicine in the community," the "community medicine model," or "*policlínicos comunitarios*."[7] The Alamar teaching clinic was the first to implement this experimental model in November 1974, which spread to five other model clinics in March 1976. By 1979, 73 percent of Cuban polyclinics had adopted the community medicine model.[8]

What appeared most important to López about this transformation was that the old *policlínico integral* had been a clinic of specialties, but they did not visit the community. By contrast,

> the *policlínico comunitario* was based on visiting people in their communities. Specialists began working together as a team. There had been many complaints that patients went to different specialists. Family medicine integrated the work of specialists.[9]

The primary teams in community medicine were composed of a physician (that is, a pediatrician, internist, or obstetrician-gynecologist) and a nurse with the same specialty. They were responsible not only for those who went to the clinic, but also for all those in their outreach territory. This special kind of outreach, which Cubans call *dispensarización,* included regular assessment-and-risk evaluation. It could be called "active medicine," because physicians did not passively wait for a patient to become ill but instead would seek out those at high risk to intervene before or just after a disease began. They would look for disorders likely to affect adolescents, women, or the elderly and were especially vigilant for indicators of hypertension, diabetes, heart disease, stroke, asthma, or tuberculosis.[10] López explained to me that physicians at the *policlínico comunitario* where he worked would use *dispensarización* to classify the health risks of patients, and after one or two visits of the patient to the clinic, the doctor would visit the patient at home.[11] Doctor-nurse teams spent about twelve hours per week doing home visits, health education, and work with community groups. Polyclinic staff was expected to work with community organizations for health education and promotion. When needed, a specialist participated in discussions between the patient and physician as a consultant.[12]

Reorganizing the clinics had a range of effects. There was much more productive interaction between specialists instead of all going their own way, as often occurred in the old model. Teamwork among medical disciplines resulted in non-physician voices challenging the dominance of physicians. The division of a clinic's service area into subsections made it easier for a chart to be retrieved from the team office rather than a centralized clinic record room. Patients also appreciated the reduction in time spent waiting.[13]

Additionally, as *policlínicos comunitarios* became the norm, there was much more emphasis on teaching at all levels, and university research became part of daily clinic operations. Previously, university teaching and research had not been truly integrated into polyclinic work. Now, students, teachers, and researchers participated regularly in clinic activity and became less separated from the lives of average Cubans.[14]

As polyclinics became teaching sites, educational curricula changed for all health care personnel. New courses, based on the concept that "health and illness are conditioned by the interaction of people, as biosocial beings, with the environment," began preparing students to work in the polyclinics.[15]

Just four years after the opening of Cuba's first *policlínico comunitario*, the World Health Organization's International Conference on Primary Health Care (PHC) met in Alma-Ata. The resulting Declaration of Alma-Ata (September 12, 1978) dovetailed with Cuban health care goals. It maintained that governments have responsibility for their citizens' health and that PHC is the key to social justice internationally: "The PHC model emphasizes health promotion and disease prevention, immunization campaigns, reproductive care, and improvements in sanitation and child/maternal health."[16] The Declaration of Alma-Ata is still described in Cuban medical texts and remembered by its practitioners.

In Cuba, "secondary health care" usually means hospital care; but it can also include brief acute care, skilled attendance during childbirth, intensive care, and use of medical technology. "Tertiary health care" in Cuba typically refers to treatment in specialized hospitals such as those for cancer, burns, cardiac problems or neurosurgery. As the structure of health care delivery changed, coinciding with the Alma-Ata perspective, the number of polyclinics increased from 161 in 1962 to 260 in 1968 and, finally, to 386 in 1980. (The number of polyclinics inched up to 442 polyclinics by 2003, showing that, although the growth rate was greatest during the transformative decades of the 1960s and 1970s, their numbers continued to slowly increase.)[17]

The growing number of polyclinics, hospitals, and medical schools brought job openings in health care professions in all parts of Cuba. Vaccination campaigns led to the eradication of malaria, diphtheria, and neonatal tetanus.[18] By 1983, after a decade of community medicine, Cuban life expectancy had increased to 73.8 years from the pre-revolutionary figure of 58.8 years.[19]

One of the biggest changes during the community medicine initiative was that, for the first time since the revolution, infant mortality began its consistent long-term decrease. After going up and down during the first years of the revolution, neonatal death rates continued to drop each decade after the 1970s.[20]

Along with improvements in clinic structure, medical education, and health indicators, Cuban medicine was also introducing important innovations. Hospitals began to employ ultrasound, CAT scanners, and the first Latin American magnetic resonance imaging (MRI) equipment. Treatment research included epidermal growth factors to help burn victims, a meningococcal meningitis B vaccine, and a computerized psychological diagnostic system. Cuban doctors also became proficient in organ transplants and limb reattachments. These are just a few of the advances that were common in the developed world but almost unheard of in poor countries like Cuba.[21]

Still, there were continuing difficulties with health care delivery during the beginning of the era of community medicine. Most of these problems reflected an inability to resolve conflicts that lingered from the first polyclinic model:

1. Biological approaches continued to be emphasized much more than psychological, social, and environmental factors, resulting in health care that was not truly comprehensive.
2. Despite the emphasis on *dispensarización*, physicians were still often reacting "passively" to symptoms rather than searching for ways to prevent illness.
3. Healthy lifestyles were not promoted vigorously enough.
4. Rather than searching for how symptoms were related to social causes, doctors continued to treat illnesses only after patients visited the clinic.
5. Medical services in teaching polyclinics continued to have a higher quality than non-teaching ones.

Other problems had arisen, including the division of family medicine into three specialties, which impeded holistic medicine; patients often going to emergency rooms for faster service; polyclinics not receiving the material resources they needed; and polyclinic patients not being adequately accompanied by polyclinic staff when hospitalized.[22]

Despite this vast array of problems, one concern permeated all others: the polyclinics still were not sufficiently a part of neighborhood and family life. Hence, health planners were searching for a modification that would bring social factors to the forefront of medical interventions, focus on lifestyle issues, and stimulate local participation in the prevention and treatment of sickness.[23]

THE FAMILY DOCTOR-NURSE PROGRAM

José Díaz Novás and José Fernández Sacasas write that "President Fidel Castro Ruz proposed the creation of a new type of medical specialty in Cuba: the family doctor. Family doctors would be charged with primary care at the neighborhood level."[24] This is the official description of the origin of family medicine. Being a bit skeptical that the entire plan for reorganization of the country's health care sprang from Fidel like Athena from the head of Zeus, I spoke with Dr. Justo

Piñeiro Fernández and Dr. Julio López Benítez about changes during that period, which both lived through. They agreed on Fidel's role. His genius was the ability to listen to ideas about medicine and translate proposals into speeches that inspired people to action.[25] Throughout the early 1980s, Cuban medical practitioners and planners intensely discussed solutions to shortcomings they experienced in polyclinics, and Fidel Castro went across the island speaking in favor of a family-doctor approach and preparing people for its inauguration.[26]

On January 4, 1984, the family doctor program—also known as "the family doctor-and-nurse team" model or the "Comprehensive General Medicine" model—began as a test project in Havana's Lawton polyclinic and quickly spread. [27] Explanations of this neighborhood system often suggest that it represented the first appearance of Cuba's doctor-nurse teams, but this was not the case. As described above, doctor-nurse teams had been an essential part of *policlínicos comunitarios*.[28] Ross Danielson published his book on the subject in 1979, years before the Lawton project. The difference was that the doctor-nurse teams in community polyclinics had been based on medical specialties, which meant that families dealt with multiple teams, each focusing on different issues. The new doctor-nurse teams, by contrast, were responsible for all medical issues and for a smaller number of patients.

Another fundamental difference is that the new teams had homes in the neighborhood they served and worked in a *consultorio* (medical office). The most typical *consultorio* was a three-family apartment retrofitted to locate the medical office on the first floor and the homes of the doctor and nurse and their families on the other two floors. Unlike other medical offices throughout the world, patients were not differentiated by income, age, or pathology. Patients were simply those who were neighbors of the health team, living in a defined geographic area.[29]

The team's proximity to its patients made it highly accessible to citizens and increased the frequency of home visits. In urban areas, the best way for doctors and nurses to make home visits was to walk to each family. Because the teams had fewer patients and lived near

them, it became possible for all Cubans to know their health practitioners well.

The geographically defined area for each doctor-nurse team would
include 120 to 150 families, or 600 to 800 individuals, within two
to three square blocks in most cities and towns.[30] The teams were
required to see every patient at least twice a year.[31] Family doctors had
a regular schedule of office hours in the morning, and made home
and field visits in the afternoon. Although the family medicine teams
worked in specific neighborhoods, they became better connected to
the medical system as a whole and were closely linked to physicians
representing fifty-four specialties.[32]

It was during the 1980s that *policlínicos comunitarios* were conceptualized, came into existence, and then evaluated and redesigned
to reflect the concepts of family medicine. Key to this process was
a novel residency program called General Comprehensive Medicine
(*Medicina General Integral*, MGI). The new family doctors were to be
very different from the old general practitioners. Medical students'
education was geared toward addressing the most frequent problems.
Courses would bring together clinical practice, hygiene, and epidemiology with clinical theory, social sciences, and biomedical sciences.[33]

The MGI program required a residency at a polyclinic with rotations at specialty hospitals. Practitioners would be thoroughly trained
in secondary and tertiary care approaches of the broader medical
system. The recently trained family practitioners committed themselves to at least five years of service in a single community. Though
the origin of the MGI program is sometimes given as 1984 or 1985,
the Cuban medical historian José R. Ruíz traces it to 1982, which is
more likely since Fidel was promoting this alternative approach from
the very early 1980s.[34] The fully developed MGI program was in place
by 1989.

How did these modifications in health care delivery and updated
curriculum affect the number of students in medical school?
Whiteford and Branch suggest that during the 1980s "attention
shifted away from how to train more medical personnel toward how
to increasingly integrate medical practice into the community and

make it part of community life."[35] However, other accounts point to a greater number of medical staff being needed to fulfill the needs of community medicine. Moreover, Kirk and Erisman document that, whereas 9,410 doctors had graduated in the 1970s, 22,490 graduated during the period 1980–89.[36] On top of that, Cuba was expanding its international medical missions during the 1980s, making it likely that more, rather than fewer, doctors were needed.

The doctor-nurse family teams were closely linked to the polyclinics and hospitals. The polyclinic would provide backup for patient care when the family doctor was unavailable. In addition to having a range of specialists in its staff, the polyclinic would keep PHC doctors updated on new procedures and serve as a training center for residents and as a clinical teaching location for professors.[37] López remembered that, after family medicine began in 1984, "there was not a big difference between doctors from *consultorios* and *policlínicos* visiting families because *consultorio* doctors were on staff at *policlínicos*."[38] *Consultorio* doctors had hospital night duties, which allowed them to visit their patients who had been hospitalized and consult with specialists for work with the patient after release.[39] Unless a patient went to a hospital distant from the *consultorio* (provincial or specialty hospital), the family doctor accompanied the patient.[40]

The family doctor program combined the advantages of small-town close relationships between doctor and patient with big-city hospital expertise. By encouraging social bonding between medical staff and patients the new system aimed to increase family participation in health care, emphasize healthy lifestyles, improve preventive care, help doctors make early diagnoses, and provide continuity of care when patients needed polyclinic or hospital attention. Health care was vastly more accessible since the doctor (or polyclinic staff) was available twenty-four hours per day. This in turn improved in-home treatment by both family members and doctors, who could be more directly involved in rehabilitation. Observing patients in their homes allowed doctors to assess the causes of illnesses more accurately than when they had relied only on patients' testimonies during office visits. In addition to addressing these relationships between patients and medical staff, the family doctor system aimed to facilitate patients' consulting with specialists at the *consultorio* and reduce delays in obtaining lab and X-ray results. The polyclinics continued to play vital roles in providing ongoing training of *consultorio* staff and as sites for teaching medical students and conducting community research.[41]

Concerns with Family Medicine

Despite what seemed to be enormous advantages of the doctor-nurse teams, agreement was not unanimous. Discord arose as the approach expanded. A team from the American Public Health Association came to Cuba in 1995 and 1996, visiting care centers without prior notification. They met many practitioners who did not accept some of the government's policies. A few expressed their lack of enthusiasm about "green medicine," which used herbs popular in Afro-Cuban culture. Others were worried about the value of "thermalism," based on mineral properties of thermal sites. As a result, MINSAP conducted research and made recommendations on using each of these methods for specific diseases.[42]

In an interview with Candace Wolf, Dr. Gilberto Fleites Gonzales voiced strong disapproval of the entire family medicine system. He heartily endorsed local polyclinics, which "did a very good job at prevention, early diagnosis and treatment" and were a "good model for primary care." Fleites also liked having "secondary care at the level of the hospitals" as well as "tertiary care, which are the institutes—the National Cancer Institute, the National Cardiology Institute, and so on." It was, according to him, "the model in the '60s, the '70s, and perfectly well established at the peak of excellency in the '80s."[43]

By contrast, Fleites had a low opinion of the new model: "Along came this idea—all physicians were against it—of the 'Block Physician.'" He claimed that the family doctor-nurse program was unnecessary and compromised the quality of care, because

> you become a physician who sees so few persons and such a limited number of cases and diseases that you end up lacking in

training. You devolve in terms of your medical training when you are the physician of one single block in the city.

Instead, Fleites advocated that the country's system focus on heart attacks and cancer, which are the number one and two causes of deaths in Cuba. Indeed, data confirm that the top five causes of death in Cuba in 1984 were heart disease, malignant tumors, cardiovascular disorders, flu, pneumonia, and accidents.[44]

Fleites did not advocate adopting a foreign model but rather defended the achievements of Cuban medicine:

> I do not look to the United States for answers. I don't like the system you have in the United States. I don't like it at all. There are many things that are very bad in the States, such as not having universal health care and the high rate of violence in your society. . . . You are on your way to destroying the earth and the peoples of the planet with your greed and your nuclear weapons.[45]

Fleites's arguments are serious ones, but they do not take into account the tremendous amount of insights that doctor-nurse teams get during home visits. Howard Waitzkin provides an example of how important this can be for the patient. He describes how, shortly after the doctor-nurse teams were established, there was a case involving a forty-year-old woman who was hospitalized due to methanol poisoning from home-brewed rum. Following discharge, the family doctor made a home visit and discovered an array of problems: safety hazards from poor home construction, an unmaintained latrine, husband/father abandonment, lack of employment, and emotional disturbances in the woman's four children.[46]

The doctor spoke with the local People's Power group, representatives of the city government, and a sanitary worker. Together, they coordinated voluntary labor to repair hazards in the home and built a toilet connected to the municipal sewer. Contacted by the doctor, a representative of the Federation of Cuban Women helped the patient get work as a hospital aide. The primary care team of doctor, nurse, and psychologist also worked with each of the four children and their schools. A teenage daughter finished school and also got a job. During a follow-up visit, the patient complained of mice in the home. The doctor noticed garbage in the yard and had sanitary workers help the patient understand the importance of trash removal.[47]

Linda Whiteford and Laurence Branch recount an interview that also underscores the importance of doctor-nurse teams making home visits. In 1993, a U.S. doctor visiting a neighborhood clinic in Matanzas was surprised at how frequently doctors see babies during their first six months of life. He thought that attending to healthy babies would take up far too much time and was even more astonished to learn that Cuban doctors visit babies in the home. A Cuban doctor in the clinic explained:

> While I am there I see the baby and mother, but I also see the grandmother, the elderly uncle, and the teenage daughter. I can see how they are feeling; I can see if the grandmother is depressed, if the daughter needs someone to talk to about birth control, if the uncle is drinking too much. And I can see how they are responding to the new baby. And because I go so often I can see if there are changes in the family over time. No, it's not excessive if I can see 5 or 6 people and help forestall problems that might deteriorate without some attention.[48]

Both the doctor attending the woman with methanol poisoning and the one visiting healthy babies show the importance of home visits. It is highly unlikely that either would have been able to respond proactively had he seen the patient in a faraway office. This is one reason that cost comparisons between preventive medicine and curative medicine are difficult to make. In effect, it is hard to calculate the money saved when preventive medicine makes future medical services unnecessary.

The essence of *dispensarización* (outreach involving assessment and risk evaluation) is observing people's behavior outside of the clinical setting. Because lifestyle patterns are critical for prevention, assessment, and rehabilitation of medical conditions, Cuban medical schools train practitioners to look closely at the relations between behavior and medical conditions.[49] This is why Cuban health care has increasingly focused on "reducing risk factors and implementing national health promotion programs such as encouraging exercise, improving diet, and reducing smoking, alcohol intake, and obesity."[50]

SOCIAL RELATIONSHIPS IN MEDICINE

In pre-revolutionary Cuba, racism affected every aspect of medicine: there were fewer hospitals in rural areas and eastern Cuba where black people predominate; mutualist clinics had many fewer black enrollees; and it was almost impossible for black people to enter medical school. By the time the family doctor system had taken root, black communities were receiving the same medical services, and Cuba was training black doctors at a rate proportional to the island's black population.[51]

The revolutionary government was always conscious of the need to increase productivity, but labor organizations checked all efforts to do so at the expense of workers' health. Raising productivity goals in the sugar industry might easily have increased the incidence of bagassosis, a chronic lung disease. However, damage from this occupational disease has been minimized by regular checkups on workers' lung functioning and efforts to reduce bagasse dust in cane processing. It is likely that health planners and sugar workers understood that short-term production gains could be offset by long-term health costs.[52]

A note about doctor-nurse teams is important for U.S. readers: Despite an increase of women doctors in the United States, male physicians still hold more powerful institutional positions and nurses are overwhelmingly female. For this reason, the phrase "doctor-nurse team" is likely to conjure up images of a male doctor working with a female nurse. This gender dyad does indeed characterize many doctor-nurse teams in Cuba. Nevertheless, women poured into medical school after the revolution and by 1970 comprised the majority of medical students.[53] Conversely, nursing has long been a mixed-gender occupation in Cuba. I saw this confirmed when I visited the Havana cemetery and saw that the old section dedicated to nurses was labeled "*Enfermeros*," the noun for nurses that means mixed gender (or all male). Had the profession been overwhelmingly female, it would have been labeled "*Enfermeras*."

While Cuban medicine has consistently sought to increase community participation, most efforts had been channeled through formal structures such as the Federation of Cuban Women, Committees for Defense of the Revolution, and local People's Power groups.[54] Family doctors and nurses living in the community was a more radical approach, which dramatically increased the opportunities for average Cubans to actively participate in health care delivery. Of course, it did not function perfectly. Several years after the introduction of community medicine, patients often were not fully involved in their own care. This has been the case even more in secondary and tertiary care institutions where "many doctors seem unaccustomed to answering questions about recommendations for procedures." Of course, interactions people have with specialists inside institutions for very serious medical problems are different from conversations in *consultorios* and *policlínicos*. [55]

Overall, medicine in the community powerfully affects the "nuances of the doctor-patient relationship," as Howard Waitzken has argued.[56] The entire training of family doctors and nurses has them focusing on environmental factors, and for that reason they do not fail to consider how personal conflicts may contribute to medical problems. The setting of patients' discussing issues in their homes rather than sitting opposite a physician in an office encourages them to be able to tell their own story with fewer interruptions. Further, since the doctors themselves are no longer only white men with an elite family tree, the patient-doctor relation takes place on a more equal footing. That Cuba promotes dialogue between doctors and patients contrasts sharply with U.S. health care, where corporate control of medicine pushes physicians to shorten conversations in order to meet patients' per-hour productivity targets.[57]

Remarkably, Cuba has been able to simultaneously develop its physical infrastructure at the same time it has redefined health care. Just as the number of polyclinics grew most rapidly in the first years after the revolution and then continued to grow more slowly; the number of hospitals doubled in the first decade of the revolution, then crept from 270 in 1984 to 281 in 2002.[58] As the structure of health care transformed, Cuba expanded secondary and tertiary care and incorporated technological innovations unknown in other poor countries.

By 1989, Cuba's official position was that "the family doctor-and-nurse model of primary care is the highest expression of the organization of primary care and of the Cuban health system as a whole. It incorporates the positive contributions of preceding models and includes new concepts."[59] It is important to highlight that this model, which has enjoyed over thirty years of permanence, is the result of decades of discussion, reassessment, and continuous tweaking. The key phases of this process can be summarized as follows:

1. For the first five years of the revolution, medicine focused on expanding care to those who had not received it.
2. During the decade beginning in 1964, medicine integrated a disparate array of services into a coherent health care system combining preventive care with treatment and providing a single point of entry (the *policlínico integral*) for every patient, based on where she or he lived.
3. In 1974, *policlínicos comunitarios* began to evaluate patients for risks, integrate the work of specialists, and transform medicine by having doctors visit patients in their homes.
4. In 1984, the first *consultorios,* each linked to a *policlínico comunitario,* significantly altered the work of doctor-nurse teams through their placement inside neighborhoods. Medical education was also transformed by developing the new MGI training program.

A superficial glance at these dates might suggest the existence of ten-year stages in the evolution of Cuban health care, but this would be a misleading oversimplification. In fact, each major change had been conceptualized, debated, and planned years before being implemented. Also, the changes in the system, whatever the date given for their formal initiation, took varying amounts of time to spread throughout the island and in the process continued to evolve. Though the Cuban model borrowed from Eastern European countries as it responded to immediate post-revolutionary crises and established its first polyclinics, it borrowed only what it chose to borrow. As López commented to me, "Public health was something we learned as we went along."[60]

— 5 —

CUBAN DOCTORS IN ANGOLA

When the Cuban health care system was implementing *policlínicos comunitarios* in the 1970s, doctors were called on to serve in an international military conflict in Angola. Taking place in the context of Portugal's internal turmoil and the loss of its colonies, for Cuba's doctors it dwarfed all its previous overseas efforts combined. It would prepare Cuban doctors to confront a possible invasion of their own country—a threat made palpable by the election of Ronald Reagan as U.S. president in 1980.

The tale is often spun that Cuba intervened in Angola first, and then, in response, the United States supported Angola's right-wing forces and the South African army accompanying them. This story is so grotesquely false that it is necessary to describe the real sequence of events leading up to Fidel's decision to participate in the struggle. In fact, after Cuba's 1967 departure from the Congo, efforts were focused on Guinea-Bissau, where Cuba saw great potential, and so did not cultivate a relationship with the Popular Movement for the Liberation of Angola (MPLA).

In April 25, 1974, Portuguese military officers and a strong popular movement overthrew the dictator, Marcello Caetano. In this new scenario, three Angolan groups began jockeying for position in the independence struggle. The MPLA, headed by doctor and poet Agostinho Neto, was the only group having even a hint of a class perspective. The National Front for the Liberation of Angola was led by Holden Roberto. Disorganized and corrupt, the FNLA's greatest strength was support from neighboring Zaire's right-wing Joseph Mobutu, who had played a central role in the assassination of Patrice Lumumba. Jona Savimbi headed the National Union for the Total Independence of Angola (UNITA). Savimbi was personally charming and spent most of his time in the field with his troops, But he had collaborated with the Portuguese during their war against the MPLA and worked hand-in-hand with the apartheid regime of South Africa.

The January 15, 1975, Alvor Agreement between the new Portuguese government and the three rebel groups set independence day as November 11, 1975. Until then, the country would be governed by a commissioner from Portugal in consultation with one representative each from the MPLA, FNLA, and UNITA. Each group had different strengths: the MPLA was the most competent and able to govern; the FNLA had the most weapons; and UNITA's Savimbi was the most adept at personal manipulation.

Angola had been the richest of Portugal's colonies, producing coffee, diamonds, iron ore, and oil. Of the former colonies, it also had the largest white population: 320,000 out of a total population of 6.4 million.[1] When 90 percent of its white population fled in 1974, Angola lost most of its skilled labor and was left with an overwhelmingly illiterate population.[2] Only fourteen doctors remained in the entire country, something that resonated with the Cuban post-revolutionary experience.[3] Moreover, the Cuban doctors who went to the Congo in 1965 had witnessed the devastating effects of losing medical professionals.[4] Still, when MPLA head Neto requested aid from Cuba in July and October 1974, Castro initially held back, recalling the consequences of having sent support to Zairean rebels based on incomplete information.[5]

For its part, the United States was initially too obsessed by the victory of Vietnam's National Liberation Front to directly intervene in Angola. Nevertheless, the CIA increased funding to the FNLA

TABLE 5.1: Contending Forces in Southern Africa

ALLIES OF CUBA AND THE SOVIET UNION	
MPLA	Popular Movement for the Liberation of Angola, founded by Agostinho Neto and later led by José Eduardo dos Santos.
FAPLA	People's Armed Forces for the Liberation of Angola, military arm of the MPLA.
ANC	African National Congress, rebels opposing racists of South Africa, sometimes trained in Angola.
ALLIES OF SOUTH AFRICA AND THE UNITED STATES	
UNITA	National Union for the Total Independence of Angola, pro-South Africa Angolans headed by Jonas Savimbi.
FNLA	National Front for the Liberation of Angola, pro-South Africa Angolans headed by Holden Roberto.

and Roberto in July 1974 and, by spring of 1975, Henry Kissinger was urging President Gerald Ford to give military aid to Savimbi.[6] Portugal had told South Africa to remove its troops from Angola, and it complied in October 1974. However, in less than a year (July 1975) South Africa was back in Angola, with encouragement from the Ford administration that lied to Congress regarding its covert military and political aid.[7] South Africa would not tolerate the MPLA's uncompromising hostility to apartheid and found willing allies in the FNLA and UNITA.

Meanwhile, Fidel's representatives met with Neto in late December 1974 along with the head of the MPLA's recently organized military wing, the Popular Armed Forces for the Liberation of Angola (FAPLA). The Angolans asked Cuba to help with training and give them $100,000 for the transport of weapons from the Soviet Union. The Cubans, however, thought that Angola would not experience civil war for two to three years, and the $100,000 came from Yugoslavia instead.[8] Clearly, Cuba was not rushing to intervene in Angola. In fact, Cuba did not commit until it became evident that Angola's antiracist government would fall without its help.

Since the FNLA controlled two northern provinces bordering Zaire, it had a steady supply line of war materials. Though the FNLA appeared to be strong, when it attacked poor areas loyal to the MPLA in the capital city of Luanda in 1975, the FAPLA defended the city with the Soviet weapons it had received. This shattered the illusion of the FNLA's invincibility.[9] Following summer talks between Cuban and Angolan leaders, three ships bearing three hundred Cuban military instructors left Havana in September and reached Angola in October. By early October 1975, it was clear that the MPLA was winning, and South Africa would either have to accept an MPLA victory or send troops. A small number of South Africans had clashed with the FAPLA on October 5, but the major South African invasion, "Operation Savannah," began on October 14. By November 4, Fidel had realized that without help the Angolan capital would fall to apartheid forces, and he decided to intervene. On November 10, there was a major battle at Quifangondo, which was the first time South Africa attacked with airplanes. Only a small number of Cubans had arrived by then, but they were critical in stopping the South African drive to Luanda. Cuba soon developed a strategy that it would pursue during the more than ten years of warfare in Angola: FAPLA would fight against Angolan enemies (the FNLA in northern provinces), while Cuban forces would concentrate on the better armed and more disciplined South Africans (then in southern Angola). By the end of 1975, Cuba had 3,500 to 4,000 troops in Angola. They were able to defend the southern part of the country against South Africa although they had fewer men and weapons.[10]

Hostility simmered between UNITA and FNLA until it boiled over on an intense Christmas Eve, 1975. UNITA won and FNLA was crumbling.[11] Cuban troops continued flowing into Angola, and numbered 36,000 by April 1976. They reached the southern border with Namibia, completely pushing out the pro-apartheid forces.[12]

A range of factors propelled Cuba to make such an enormous investment in Angola. Often forgotten is Cuba's long history of international solidarity. In 1936–39 almost one thousand Cubans had volunteered in Spain to protect it from Francisco Franco's fascist rise to power.[13] Cuban medical students and physicians had quarreled among themselves as early as 1925 over the need to extend the medical revolution to the poorest parts of the island.[14] The 1959 revolution was immediately opposed by Eisenhower. Moreover, Kennedy's foolhardy toying with nuclear war made it clear that the revolutionary government had genuine concerns for the country's safety. Despite its toning down of revolutionary rhetoric and accommodation to the Soviets in the 1970s, it remained clear that the best defense of Cuba from the United States would be an offense. An offense in Africa would be vastly less likely to provoke a direct confrontation, largely because most Americans did not see Africa as part of its backyard. Additionally, a huge number of Cubans are of African descent and those of European descent have often seen anti-racism as core to their politics. Fidel referred to the anti-apartheid struggle as "the most beautiful cause."[15]

WHAT CUBAN DOCTORS SAW IN ANGOLA

Beginning in 1975, many Cuban doctors were not able to participate in the reconfiguration of polyclinics inside Cuba. Cuban doctors had worked to extend medical care throughout the island in the 1960s; now they were changing the lives of Angolans in the 1970s. When a Cuban medical team reached Angola's second-largest city of Huambo in March 1976, only one doctor remained there. That doctor left three months later, but the Cubans stayed. Even a local paper that disliked Castro recognized that the city lived in fear that the Cuban doctors might leave.[16]

When Hedelberto López interviewed doctors who went to Zaire, the Congo, and Guinea-Bissau in the 1960s, they recalled working in the context of the war and helping civilians. By contrast, the stories of doctors who served in Angola from 1975 to 1976 were much more focused on military injuries. The doctors who went there saw a face of war they had never witnessed before.[17]

The first Cuban doctor to arrive in Angola was Abigaíl Dambai Torres. While completing a specialty in internal medicine, he agreed to participate in an international mission but was not told where he would go. Dambai arrived in Angola in September 1975 and was assigned to the northern front where Roberto's advancing FNLA was trying to reach Luanda before independence day of November 11. They were attacked on October 23, and Dr. Dambai's first patient had serious chest and abdominal wounds from mortar fragments. Soon he had three other multi-trauma victims, one with a bullet wound that almost ripped off his arm. As enemy shells were landing next to his medical post, he prepared for a rapid evacuation. An officer told him to drop to the ground because mortar shells were landing just 250 meters away. Together they crawled for twenty minutes and then ran zigzag to avoid being shot. They reached the battalion commander and learned that another doctor had not shown up after his medical post had been bombed.

Less than three weeks later, Dambai witnessed the decisive Battle of Quifangondo, twenty-four hours before Independence Day. Aided by Cuban Special Forces, the FAPLA defeated the FNLA. As Angolan troops pursued the FNLA in the direction of Zaire, Dr. Dambai passed by the battlefield. As a physician, he had to help cleanse the area, which resembled a cemetery. "It was a horrible scene with a huge number of inflated bodies floating in the river." He stayed for a month near Quifangondo, where he treated people with wounds from mines, wounds with and without fractures, and cerebral contusions.[18]

While pursuing FNLA forces, a FAPLA truck hit a mine and blew up its gas tank, causing a death and sixteen injuries including exposed broken bones, serious burns, and a nearly severed leg. As the only physician with the necessary skills, Dambai had to cope with all the wounds himself on the ground, in the open air, under the intense African sun. The same day, he was called upon to treat fifteen victims whose vehicle had hit a mine and were then ambushed. As night approached, Dambai had to work under truck headlights so he could treat all the patients lying on the ground, prevent shock, do an amputation, and attend to fractures and eye traumas, all without serum. He and his medical assistants could not sleep that night, as they attended to the injured—changing bandages, adjusting tourniquets, ensuring immmobilizations, stopping the flow of blood, and alleviating pain with medications.[19]

They finally arranged to transport patients to a nearby town. Exhausted, the doctor and assistant planned to sleep during the jeep ride to Luanda. However, after going five hundred meters, the jeep oveturned and the Cuban driver stopped breathing due to cranial trauma. They put the driver in a larger jeep, which had space to continue efforts at revival, and continued on their way, hoping not to hit a mine. The injured driver finally responded, and later recovered in a Luanda hospital. When Dambai was in Quibocolo on January 24, 1976, he treated a couple of white mercenaries fighting for South Africa; an Argentinian in shock with blood flowing from an open wound to the right tibula; and a Portuguese with a right femur broken by a bullet. Angolan troops then brought in four more wounded mercenaries and another two later that night.[20]

Reflecting on the injuries he treated in thirty battles, Dambai concluded that "most of those I treated had lower body injuries from mines, which were the weapons that produced the most damage to troops." The vast area covered by the war meant that "the injured often had a long trip" to a hospital. The intensity of the war left the doctors little time to attend to civilians, but during the end of his mission Dambai was in the village of Mama Rosa where the "most frequent sicknesses were malaria, anemia, malnutrition and parasites." Later, he was asked to help in the main hospital in Luanda, where he saw over a hundred patients per day. Dambai had lost over twenty pounds by the time he returned to Cuba.[21]

Another Cuban doctor whom Hedelberto López interviewed was Pedro Luis Pedroso Fernández. Pedroso had been expelled from school for working with revolutionary students and then went to work for the telephone company. Hearing Fidel speak of the need for doctors, he began to study pre-medicine in 1962, finished his medical degree in 1969, and, after doing Rural Medical Service, returned to complete a specialty in urology in 1974. A year later, Pedroso was asked if he would participate in an international medical mission and he immediately agreed. But he did not find out where he was going until meeting with Fidel and Raúl, who made sure that everyone in his group had watches.

Pedroso reached Angola on October 5, 1975, and was stationed near the port of Benguela where his battalion was attacked by South Africans on November 3. His anesthesiologist was injured, so he had to fulfill that role as well. During the battle, Pedroso treated a captured mercenary whose leg had been blown off. He wrapped the stump and then went to deliver a baby. Pedroso later went to Quiculungo, where an ambulance driver had a leg blown off. He had brought tweezers, needles, a stethoscope, and a handsaw to use in surgery. The handsaw proved necessary for an amputation that saved the driver's life. After going south to Quibala, he did three more amputations.[22] When in the eastern city of Conde, accompanying Cuban special troops, he confronted a particularly difficult situation:

> A torrential rain began and a truck without railing arrived with thirty wounded, almost all Angolan. The torrent increased in intensity. The truck was dripping blood in a Dantesque scene. I began to treat those in the worse condition. I had four uniforms and a blanket in my backpack and put them on those who were the coldest. I buried three Angolans by the house where we were, operated on one with an abdominal wound, and treated the others.[23]

Pedroso operated on the floor of the hut with the help of an Angolan. Inside the hut, they heard the sounds of Cuban trucks going by. "Then we heard distinct motors, that did not seem to be ours. We told those with injuries to speak in a soft tone so they would not hear us. We used three containers of morphine to calm those in the most pain."[24]

They were not discovered, and Pedroso's group returned to Quibala where he was the only doctor and spent most of his time with civilian patients. Pedroso encountered "lots of cases of tuberculosis with hemoptysis, malaria, and another sickness where people had balls in their skin that disappeared in three hours." He also delivered several babies and buried a friend. His range of responsibilities went far beyond his specialty in urology:

> I had to do everything: bury, treat, and help people escape. Since I knew that battle was approaching, at different hours of the day I explored routes of evacuation for those in the hospital who had been injured. Everything was organized. Luckily, we did not leave anyone and we were able to evacuate all of the injured.[25]

He recalled a most unusual experience during the battle of Morro de Tongo. Pedroso was treating a Cuban who was about forty-eight years old for a leg wound. "As I was treating him another patient arrived. When the two were parallel to each other and I looked at them, I could see that they were father and son." Each had been recruited by a different unit and did not know that the other was in Angola. Both told him to treat the other first. "I told them that I had to treat the one who was most in need first. The son had the more severe leg wound, but I was able to attend to it and evacuate both together." Pedroso was struck by the ideological strength of the Cuban combatants. Despite the horrors of war, none of the Cubans he tried to evacuate wanted to go. "Some swore at me and one said that he was going on a hunger strike."[26] He later apologized.

Pedroso remembered that the doctors had to keep medicines for the troops and could not spare much for villagers. The reactions of the Angolans they encountered as they went from village to village was moving:

> Many people were content only to look at the medicines we had, or for us to put the stethoscope on them. The times that moved me the most was when people knelt as if I was a god; they kissed my hand, and I never forgot them. I thought that they had been neglected their entire lives and had never been seen by a doctor in the forest.[27]

Another episode that stands out in his memories:

I will never forget the beautiful little boy of about seven years who was hit by a shell fragment in Quibala. I operated and dealt with the intestinal perforations he had, but there was not enough blood to replace what he lost and he died. The face of this boy is still reflected in my eyes. It is the face of war, and therefore I am always dedicated to peace.[28]

Pedroso left Angola at the end of June in 1976. He returned for a three-month mission in 1983. When near the airport someone shouted "Doctor, Doctor!"—it was the combatant whose leg he had amputated. "I had not forgotten him since the operating conditions were not easy and his face showed such anxiety and pain. I had to use morphine even though I only had four or five containers of it. After our greeting, he hugged me and cried."[29]

Hedelberto López also interviewed Omar Prudencio Martínez Herrera, who had participated in the 1959 literacy campaign, entered medical school in October 1962 during the Missile Crisis, and graduated in 1972 as an anesthesiologist. In early December 1975, Martínez left for Angola, where he treated "everyone, Angolans, Cubans and even the enemy." From his very first days there, Martínez worked with young Angolans to prepare them to help with anesthesia, medical care, and watching over the patients. The Cubans taught classes that were both theoretical and practical:

Students learned directly in an accelerated process because there was not much time for us to have the luxury of teaching in a classroom. They had to be prepared at any hour of the day, at any moment, and in whatever quantity those with serious injuries from accidents or combatant activities arrived. At the beginning, I had to handle all of the needs of the injured. After several months, the Angolans were a great help, because they took blood pressure and pulse and watched over the patients.[30]

Like other Cuban physicians in Angola, Martínez remembered "injuries that I had never observed before. . . . There were days when we had to operate on ten to fifteen orthopedic patients in addition to those injured from guns, grenades, anti-personnel weapons, accidents, burns, which is to say, all types of injuries." He observed a similar pattern of injuries as the others: "This war was characterized by [injuries to] lower body parts and amputations." Long, exhausting hours were not unusual. "Work began at 7:30 in the morning and we finished at 8:00 at night with only short rests to eat in the same room. . . . Many times I stayed in the operating room twenty-four hours straight because I was the only anesthesiologist."[31]

Martínez observed physiological differences between Cubans and Angolans:

We had to get used to working with an extraordinary deficit of blood because a large part of the country suffered from malaria, a sickness endemic to many regions of Africa, and therefore would not risk introducing the virus to other patients. Additionally, the Cuban body is not prepared to confront the disease. When we operated on an Angolan we had only four grams of hemoglobin and they were able to recuperate fine. Low levels of hemoglobin in blood is a characteristic of many regions of Africa, very different from Cubans who required twelve grams.[32]

He was in for repeated surprises: "Since I have very black skin, some thought that I was Angolan and asked to be cared for by a Cuban. I realized that I was offering my services in a country that, in spite of its riches, was very poor." Many cases stuck in his mind, such as when he had to amputate both legs of a man due to a mine explosion, and treating the wounds of a military group that had played soccer with a grenade.[33] However, an incident that had the biggest impact was when a sapper, a combat engineer who clears minefields, had an anti-tank mine explode: "The explosion ripped off both his arms and a leg; he lost his eyes; and had multiple wounds and burns. For this reason, I often repeat that people talk about war without really knowing the enormous tragedies and horrors that its victims suffer."[34]

Martínez returned to Cuba in August 1976 and became an anesthesiologist at Carlos J. Finlay Hospital in Havana.

THE SECOND PHASE OF THE WAR

Cuba had planned to withdraw all troops from Angola during the period 1976–78 leaving only military instructors behind, and the number of its soldiers in Angola dropped from 36.000 in April 1976 to under 24,000 within a year. However, in 1977 and 1978, Katangan soldiers who had fled from Mobutu's regime in Zaire to live in Angola attacked the Zairean province of Shaba. Both times they did this without knowledge or support of Cuba. When France and Belgium sent troops to support Zaire, Cuba halted its troop withdrawal.[35]

Almost immediately after South Africa withdrew its forces from Angola in December 1975, it began to clandestinely send in troops who pretended to be part of UNITA. These included whites who blackened their faces with "Black Is Beautiful" camouflage cream. Then, on May 4, 1978, South African planes launched a major air strike inside Angola at the Cassinga camp for Namibian refuges. The raid killed sixteen Cubans and six hundred Namibians. Namibia, which was formerly German Southwest Africa and lies between South Africa and Angola, had become a South African mandate following the First World War. In 1971, the International Court of Justice ordered South Africa to withdraw from Namibia because its continuing rule was illegal. Throughout the fifteen-year Angolan conflict, South Africa and the United States studiously ignored international law and acted as if it was perfectly natural for South Africa to continue dominating Namibia. After the Cassinga massacre, U.S. president Jimmy Carter brushed it aside as a retaliatory strike against Namibian rebels and quipped that "We hope it's all over." The U.S. refusal to take any actions against the violation of Angola's national sovereignty gave a green light to South Africa to invade at will.[36]

South Africa launched another attack inside Angola in March 1979. It did so again in 1980, this time 180 kilometers deep into Angola. Encouraged by Ronald Reagan's election to the White House in 1980,

South Africa stepped up its raids, not only in Angola, but also in Mozambique, Zimbabwe, Zambia, Lesotho, Swaziland, and Botswana. On August 25, 1981, South Africa poured four to five thousand troops into southern Angola, together with tanks and air support. Later, silently backed by Washington, South Africa expanded its tactics to include poisoning wells, killing livestock, and destroying food distribution and communications. On August 14, 1983, the South African air force went so far as to attack 500 kilometers north of the Namibian border and destroyed the Angolan town of Cangama. FAPLA fell back and UNITA occupied what was left of Cangama. It was in this context that Cuba sent 9,000 troops back to Angola during August 1983.[37]

Savimbi's Pact with Racism

Throughout the Carter administration and the early Reagan years, the United States increased its flow of weapons to UNITA. By 1984, UNITA had about 36,000 soldiers compared to FAPLA's almost 50,000. As early as 1974 UNITA's leader, Savimbi, established contacts with the Portuguese dictatorship and promised South Africa that he would prevent Namibian rebels from entering Angola, while helping them build an anti-communist bloc. Savimbi spoke fluent English, oozed self-confidence, was unscrupulous, cleverly manipulated his audiences, and knew just what people in the United States wanted to hear. In other words, his combination of qualities was a perfect fit for a CIA front man. Even Lane Kirkland invited Savimbi to speak to the AFL-CIO in 1979.[38] Acting as a cult leader, he had total power in UNITA and did not tolerate dissent. By 1980, in addition to ridding UNITA of those who challenged him, Savimbi had "the wives and children of the dissenters burned alive in public displays to teach the others."[39] In contrast to the Cuban practice of incorporating traditional healers into the medical system, Savimbi executed village opponents as "sorcerers" as a way of consolidating his power.

UNITA was not only a threat to Angolan and Cuban troops, but also to Cuban aid workers, including medical professionals. Even the *New York Times*, which habitually overlooked Savimbi's brutality, pointed out in 1984 that UNITA had "targeted Cuban workers for kidnapping and assassination." Dr. Oscar Mena Hector was in Luanda for eight months in the period 1977–78. He and other physicians lived under the shadow of UNITA's offer of "$10 for every Cuban head cut off and given to them, whether military or doctor." Four doctors he knew went to the front and two died there.[40]

Savimbi was key to South Africa's political strategists. Special Forces Colonel Jan Breytenbach saw Savimbi as a "manipulator extraordinaire. . . . As a political leader, he was very good. I would compare him to Hitler." (In South Africa's racist political context, this comparison to Hitler was meant as a compliment, as multiple top South African politicians had been members of pro-Nazi groups.) Savimbi returned the South Africans' admiration. When P. W. Botha was inaugurated as South Africa's first executive president, the boycott by the international community was so widespread that even Pinochet's Chile and Israel took part (despite the latter having sold arms to the apartheid regime). Yet Savimbi was one of five black politicians who attended. The fantasy of a well-educated anti-communist guerrilla leader proved seductive to the corporate press, and false stories circulated that Savimbi had a PhD from the University of Lausanne, leading South African politicians to refer to him as "Dr. Savimbi."[41]

Successive U.S. administrations admired him. Among those who overlooked Savimbi's campaigns of mass destruction and murder was President Jimmy Carter, who took time out from his human rights advocacy to arrange for secret financing of UNITA. Ronald Reagan, as rabidly anti-Castro as John and Robert Kennedy had been, had no qualms about working with Savimbi. In 1985, Steve Weissman, of the House Foreign Affairs Subcommittee on Africa, explained the bipartisan stance: "We wanted to hurt Cuba, and we wanted to help people who wanted to hurt Cuba. When Savimbi said that he was 'fighting for freedom against Cuba' this was his trump card. It was impossible to counter it. Savimbi had one redeeming quality: he killed Cubans."[42]

South African attitudes toward Savimbi fit into its broader perspective of utter contempt for blacks.. When South Africa's Breytenbach first began to organize FNLA recruits in 1975, he wrote back: "I stared distastefully and with sick foreboding at the most miserable, under-fed, ragged and villainous bunch of troops I had ever seen in my life." His attitude paralleled the treatment of black soldiers in the South African military. Its Buffalo Battalion had white officers command-ing black soldiers. Deaths of whites were followed by announcements from the army and obituaries in the press, while deaths of black sol-diers were kept silent. Deaths of black soldiers were not broadcast by either their military superiors or by the press at home.[43]

South African policy coincided with that of the United States. When the world imposed economic sanctions on South Africa, a 1971 amendment to the U.S. sanctions bill introduced by former KKK member Senator Robert Byrd (D-WV) exempted chrome imports, thereby lessening consequences to the white minority government of Rhodesia. As anti-apartheid protests mounted, Ronald Reagan's assis-tant secretary for Africa, Chester Crocker, showed his allegiances by empathizing with what he called "the awesome political dilemma in which Afrikaners and other whites find themselves." In 1986, Reagan himself notoriously lavished praise on South African whites, saying they gave great opportunities to blacks.[44]

Sophia Ndeitungo, a survivor of the South African massacre at the refugee camp in Cassinga, vividly remembered the Cubans who came to rescue them. Since the rescuers were mostly white, the twelve-year-old Namibian girl thought they were South Africans. "Later, we understood that not all whites are bad." After the massacre, Sophia was relocated to Cuba's Isle of Youth to study far away from bombs of South Africa. She graduated from medical school in Havana, married another Cassingan refugee, and returned to Namibia to become head of its armed forces medical services in 2007. For thousands of black Africans, Cuban doctors and soldiers were the only white people who showed them any kindness.[45]

Cuban Missions in Angola

After Angola won its independence in 1975, Cubans sought to fill the void produced by the flight of Portuguese skilled labor and professionals. They helped rebuild roads and railroads, supervised port operations and coordinated airport and communication facilities. By 1978, almost 7,000 aid workers were in Angola. Construction workers, teachers, and health staff comprised the largest groups. In Cuba, a new generation had come of age, schooled to help others, including via international aid. Although political enthusiasm was a motivator, everyone knew that service in Angola would look good on a job application upon returning to Cuba. The few who were reluctant to join an international mission might feel pressure from friends and family, and a member of the Communist Youth who declined a mission invitation could expect any future career in the Party to vanish. It should be remembered that this was a time when many U.S. citizens had to flee to Canada to escape being drafted for the Vietnam War. By contrast, Cubans refusing to go to Angola were not forced to flee to another country to avoid prison.[46] The war was just one of the challenges that Cubans faced in Angola. Daily life and the tasks of humanitarian assistance were not easy. In Sumbe, one hundred construction workers were idle due to lack of materials. Schoolteachers sometimes discovered that there were no pens, books, or paper for children. Housing and work facilities could be uncomfortable, since the war left many buildings in disrepair. Food was available, but it was not always the best. One aid worker recalled eating sardines from Cuba day after day. Others had a monotonous diet of Spam from the Netherlands: "We ended up hating it. . . . We ate Spam for lunch, dinner, it was never-ending."[47]

The Cubans who left the biggest impression on Angolans were the doctors. When Raúl Castro first told President Neto of Cuba's intention to withdraw its forces in 1976, the latter accepted it, but with the request that "the Cuban doctors remain and continue their valuable services."[48] Doctors were among those most enthusiastic to go to Angola. Dr. Oscar Mena, who attended medical school in Havana from 1970 to 1976, told me that during his graduation,

a government representative asked if anyone would volunteer to go on international missions to Africa and 100 percent of the graduating class's hands went up. Those who went to medical school in Cuba had a very strong sense both of helping everyone in Cuba and helping internationally. All eight hundred graduates went to one of several African countries where we saw many tropical diseases that we did not see in Cuba, such as [the parasitic diseases] sleeping sickness, schistosomiasis and filcetriasis. Every student spent six months studying tropical diseases and English, French, or Portuguese.[49]

Mena estimates that there were 280 Cuban doctors in Angola, from 1977 to 1978 when he was there, though Piero Gleijeses gives a figure of 324 in 1978 and 336 in 1979. One of nineteen doctors in Luanda, Mena worked five days per week, saw thirty to forty children every morning, and did internal medicine with more than thirty adults each afternoon. On Sundays, his group took a bus through the jungle to vaccinate children in rural areas.[50]

Dr. Carlos Suárez Monteagudo attended medical school from 1969 to 1976 and then did social service for five years before serving in Angola as a general practitioner from December 1981 through November 1983. He had wanted to go to Ethiopia in 1978 but was told he needed to complete his social service before participating in an overseas mission. When I asked if all medical students accepted doing social service, he responded, "Yes, because it was part of becoming a doctor."

In Angola, Suárez was first in the capital city of Luanda. UNITA did not attack the city, but the military brought patients with gunshot wounds and other war injuries from the front to the civilian hospital where he worked. The Cuban medical staff also provided free care to Angolans for problems such as malaria, tropical diseases, tuberculosis, and leprosy.[51] There was no electricity where he lived, and there usually was none at the hospital. The only electricity came from generators, but sometimes doctors had to perform surgery even without it. Water was also precarious, being brought in by trucks. Although elective surgery could be postponed until water was restored, the doctors sometimes had to perform emergency surgery without it.

When Suárez was transferred to Moxico province, his group was in an isolated location where there was often insufficient food. When there was food, it tended to be repetitive. Suárez lost forty-five pounds the first year he was in Angola. With anemia and starvation abundant in the country, Angolan children frequently had iron levels that were too low for operations. Cuban doctors often gave their own blood to these children so they could perform the surgery. Suárez felt that Cubans developed good relationships with the Angolan people. He trained Angolan nurses in hygiene, anatomy, physiology, and use of basic medical equipment. After returning to Cuba, Suárez completed his specialty in neurology, was part of the group that founded the Centro Internacional de Restauración Neurológica, working there as a subdirector for nine years, and then served as its director for twenty-three years.[52]

Dr. Jorge Luís Martínez and Dr. Angel Chang explained to me how Cuba *influenced* but did not *transform* the Angolan medical system. For example, Cuba did not create *policlínicos comunitarios* or promote family medicine there. Not finding a primary health care system in place, Martínez worked to promote preventive medicine. As an epidemiologist, he was assigned to controlling a malaria epidemic in Luanda, brought on in part by heavy rains, during the period 1984–85. He worked closely with the very few Angolan epidemiologists there. His team pursued several methods of malaria control, not only treating individuals but also destroying mosquito habitats. They also taught preventive medicine to Luandan health authorities and other people, including how to stop contamination by draining water and burning or burying garbage.[53]

Dr. Lourdes Franco Codinach was working in a Havana hospital when an administrator asked if she would go to Angola. The thirty-two-year-old physician initially hesitated, because she was divorced and living with her mother and four-year-old son. In the end, however, she decided to go where she was most needed and boarded a plane for Angola along with 162 other health care workers. When she arrived, Franco served in the medical brigade in the coastal city of Benguela, roughly midway between Luanda and the Namibian border. At that time, most aid workers went to provincial capitals. The vast majority of aid workers were either medical staff, teachers, or construction workers, with each group having its own residential building. The five-story building she lived in was large enough for everyone to have a separate bedroom. They could buy their own groceries at a building commissary and fix their own meals. Every Angolan town had an open-air market called the *candonga* where Cubans were not supposed to go for their own safety. They went on weekends anyway, and on Sundays they only went in groups, because it was more dangerous when fewer Angolans were shopping.[54]

Aid workers typically stayed for two years and had a one-month vacation in Cuba after the first eleven months. All had the right to return to their jobs upon completion of their missions. When Franco went to Angola, the average medical brigade was half women; it had twenty-eight members with sixteen of them being doctors. In Benguela, the only other medical personnel were Soviet citizens (five doctors and a nurse) and Angolans (two doctors and a few nurses). Franco worked in the Benguela hospital, taught a pediatric medical class to Angolan nurses, and made a weekly trip to treat rural patients. When in school, she had been turned down from joining the communist youth organization because she was a practicing Catholic (not permitted in the Party at that time). She was made acting brigade head during her last three weeks in Angola and felt that not being a member of the Communist Party did not affect her work there at all. In Angola, Franco regularly attended mass on Sunday mornings and occasionally went to the local priest's house for lunch, dinner, or a party.[55]

Each week a suitcase with mail from Cuba arrived, which was important to Franco because she deeply missed her mother and son. As her two-year mission drew to a close, she received the Medal of the International Worker with other members of her medical brigade. Franco wrote her mother:

There aren't words to express everything I felt when they pinned the medal on me. It has been a great day, full of emotions and of a truth I will never forget. This medal belongs also to you because you have helped me to accomplish my duty and you have supported me through it all. The medal represents the happy culmination of this time, when I've offered my labor to these people who are in such need.[56]

Previously, she had written to soothe her mother's fears: "We are fine, although this is a country at war. The possibility of dying is present everywhere, and we are all aware of this, but here in the city there are no difficulties. ... You always think that we're in the middle of flying bullets, but this is not so." Franco may have been understating the dangers. In fact, there were increased attacks from UNITA at that time resulting in intense training of the Cuban aid workers by military personnel.[57]

North of Benguela province where Dr. Franco served was the town of Sumbe, which was even farther from the southern parts of Angola controlled by UNITA. It had been considered safe, so there were no Cuban soldiers and only three hundred Angolan militia stationed there. On March 25, 1984, more than a thousand UNITA troops swarmed into Sumbe with the goal of freeing prisoners and kidnapping Angolan government workers and foreign aid workers. Those workers included a few from Italy and Portugal, 4 Bulgarians, 38 Soviets. and 230 Cubans. Somehow, they held off UNITA for three hours until Cuban planes arrived. After a few more hours Cuban troops arrived and UNITA withdrew. The battle cost the lives of three Cuban teachers and four Cuban construction workers. The Cuban command then intensified military training of aid workers and withdrew those in isolated locations. Nevertheless, the following month, on April 19, 1984, UNITA bombed a car next to a Cuban aid workers' residence in Huambo, Angola's second-largest city, killing or wounding forty Angolans and seventy-eight Cubans.[58]

Though critical of creating neighborhood doctor-nurse teams, Dr. Gilberto Fleites Gonzalez was highly supportive of his government's efforts in Angola, where he served from 1986 to 1988:

1986 was a period of relative economic buoyancy in Cuba—with the big subsidy from the Soviet Union we could live okay. . . . All of a sudden I was sent to a country where people do not have a proper water supply—where malaria, cholera, typhoid fever are a daily issue— where life expectancy at birth is a disaster . . .

So I had to learn a whole new medicine. I had to learn about malnutrition, about malaria, typhoid fever, all the parasitic diseases. I had to learn about gunshot wounds. In Cuba I had never, ever before treated a gunshot wound patient because Cuba, being such a peaceful country, has no weapons in the hands of the population. . . . Every day, 50 percent of my practice in the emergency room in my civilian hospital were casualties of war: farmers who stepped on mines, civilians who had weapons in their house, civilians who were victims of the UNITA forces attacking their village . . . and raping and killing, stray bullets in the hands, faces, you name it. The UNITA forces . . . were quite horrible in doing a lot of damage to the population. . . . Women farming, stepping on a mine and losing one leg and the kid she was carrying on her back being hurt by the shrapnel of the mine.

One day an epidemic of cholera broke out in the forest region of the country. A team of 15 epidemiologists was sent to fight the epidemic and they needed a surgeon to accompany them into the jungle. . . . So I was sent with them. It was an amazing experience, working by the banks of the Congo River, surrounded by huge baobab trees. . . . We had a glimpse of what the continent was like before the Europeans arrived and ruined it.

He felt that he came back changed from the overseas mission:

I can truly say that my mission in Angola was one of the highlights in my life. I became a better human being by being exposed to those realities of a very poor country. I became way, way more mature in terms of understanding society and politics and armed conflicts. . . .

One of the important factors that led me into becoming an environmentalist was seeing the environmental destruction in Angola. My experience there also led me into my involvement in the prevention of nuclear war. . . . In Angola, I saw with my own eyes the destruction of a society being torn apart by civil war. I saw a society where weapons were in the hands of everybody—where men, women and children lost legs, arms, hands and fingers on a daily basis. So I think that was one of the things that led me in the direction of being an activist . . . and participating in conferences here and abroad, presenting the Cuban perspective.[59]

These are just some of the memories of battlefield medicine, community medicine, daily life in Angola, and the dangers of working there, which Cubans would later share with their families, friends, and co-workers at home. Their memories also played a role in Cuba's medical education, since students would learn about international health work directly from instructors who had served overseas.

CONFLICTS BETWEEN ALLIES

The guiding principle in U.S. policy toward Angola was what Piero Gleijeses calls "one-sided detente." This was the unspoken doctrine that the United States and its allies could protect business interests by sending troops anywhere at any time—no matter how minor the concern—but those opposing Western corporate power were denied the same right. According to this policy, the United States could send its military to Djibouti, Zaire, and countries throughout Latin America, but Cuba could not deploy troops in Angola, even if they were critical in defending Angola from a South African onslaught.

The United States' single overriding concern was to get Cuban troops out of Africa. To achieve this end, it was prepared to tolerate even a revolutionary government in Angola and a victory in Namibia of forces hostile to South Africa. Both the United States and South Africa wanted Savimbi in power in Angola and Namibia controlled by

South Africa. However, for the United States these were *preferences*, whereas for South Africa they were *requirements*. This discrepancy in priorities led to friction between the two allies, which left South Africans bitter, feeling that the United States was abandoning them.[60] By far, the greatest discord between allies arose from the marriage of necessity between Cuba and the Soviet Union, a relationship that brought ecstasy to neither partner. Since 1975, Cuba's strategy in Angola had been for it to confront the better-armed and better-trained South African forces, while Angola's FAPLA would confront internal enemies through guerrilla warfare. By contrast, the Soviets believed that FAPLA should develop a conventional army, with tanks and heavy weapons, to fight South Africa. Moscow did not attribute much importance to internal enemies. As UNITA replaced FNLA as the primary enemy, Cuba continued to advocate that the FAPLA should focus on the constantly moving targets as it was experienced doing while the Soviets thought that victory would stem from a more conventional military strategy, based on capturing the enemy's capital. President Neto agreed with the Cubans that FAPLA lacked the organization and discipline to confront South Africa. At least as important was the Angolan troops' lack of formal education. Officers might have reached the second, third, or fourth grade, but the army's rank and file typically had never been to school and were unable to master the sophisticated weapons provided by the Soviets.[61] As the fighting became more bloody, Cuba cautioned that the Angolan military should have Cuban backup whenever venturing into territory replete with UNITA and South African troops. President Neto died in September 1979, and his successor, José Eduardo dos Santos, was often lured by Soviet visions of having a conventional army strong enough to overcome both internal and external enemies. However, this strategy led to Angolan defeats at Carreira (1979), Cuangar (1980), Mavinga (1980), and Cuvelai (1984).[62] Throughout the conflict, the Soviets acted as if the primary weapons of war were logistical plans, tanks, and weapons, whereas for Cuba the maps of war were drawn from the hearts and minds of those who used the materièl. This meant that Cuba understood that the Angolan war was part of a broad campaign against racist domination across southern Africa. While the Soviets minimized the anti-apartheid struggle as something that would "take a long time," Fidel watched it with an eagle's eye, considering it valuable in and of itself and capable of weakening South Africa's expeditionary force.[63] Cuba's initial victory over South Africa in 1976 let loose a "tidal wave" against white racist rule as black Africans in the whole region perceived the vulnerability of the apartheid forces. Mozambique became independent, and a few months later demonstrations erupted in Soweto, South Africa. In September 1977 black leader Steve Biko died in police custody and within a month the government had banned 18 organizations and the most important black newspaper. By the late 1970s Cuba had provided guerrilla training to over one hundred South Africans who fled to Angola. When, in 1984, a new South African constitution bestowed political participation upon "Coloreds" and Indians but denied the same rights to blacks, black townships in the industrial centers of the country exploded. Massive demonstrations, strikes, school walkouts, and boycotts of white-owned stores spread like wildfire. Funerals for victims of state repression became important sites of protest. The ceremony for awarding the Nobel Peace Prize to Bishop Desmond Tutu drew a huge rally. Internal and external opposition to apartheid expanded simultaneously with the intensification of the Angolan war. By 1987 the South African demonstrations were so large that thousands of white soldiers were assisting police within its borders. In 1988, a massive school walkout found miners striking in solidarity.[64] Fidel understood how these events figured into the Angolan war strategy in a way that the Soviets seemed unable to grasp.

A cultural gap between Cubans and Soviets morphed into another military difference between the allies. When reminiscing about the Academy for Senior Officers, an Angolan general noted: "We had only Soviet professors, but they weren't very knowledgeable about guerrilla warfare and they hadn't adjusted to life in Africa." Soviet personnel were generally aloof around those they came to help and seemed to see their assistance as merely a job. By contrast, Cuban soldiers and doctors blended into Angolan society. During the period 1976–77, Cubans were training young anti-apartheid recruits of the African National Congress at Novo Catengue, Angola. One recruit remembered that the "Cubans ate what we ate, slept in tents like us, lived as we did." Dr. Franco, who frequently dined with her Angolan friends, made a similar observation when she wrote from Benguela: "[The Soviets] don't make friends with Angolans. They don't socialize with them like we do." Battlefields reflected this cultural chasm—Soviet advisers stood on the sidelines while Cubans always joined in combat.[65]

In 1985, the contrast between Cuban and Soviet strategies sharpened. The Cubans had long believed that they should be the force directly confronting South African troops. Now, with the rapidly expanding anti-apartheid confrontations and serious military blunders by the Soviets, Fidel believed that the time had come for Cuba to directly attack South African forces and drive them out of Angola. The Soviets were aghast at this idea.

Despite their opposing interpretations and frequent arguments, the Cubans and Soviets came together in their opposition to Angola negotiating with South Africa and the United States behind their backs. When the Angolans listened to Cuba, they tended to agree that they could not go it alone against South Africa and should concentrate on guerrilla combat with UNITA. But the Soviets repeatedly lured them with promises of a quick resolution of the war if they would strike aggressively in a way that Cuba deemed foolish. Most likely, this was in part a response to the tug-of-war between Cuba and the Soviet Union over strategy. Usually, the Angolans would inform their allies following discussions, but often they did not tell their war partners what happened. Since the Soviets were footing the bill for the entire military effort and Cuba was witnessing a rising toll of death and injury among its soldiers and aid workers, they shared a frustration with Angola, which sometimes brought them closer together.

CUBA'S INTERNATIONAL MISSIONS

Before 1975, fewer than two thousand Cubans had been on medical, military, or other missions. During the Angolan conflict, Cuban international missions—especially medical missions to Africa—grew by leaps and bounds. Before that time, doctors had accompanied military missions to Zaire, the Congo, Guinea-Bissau, Sierra Leone, and Somalia. By the end of the 1980s Cuban aid had reached more than a dozen African countries. These included Benin, Burkina Faso, Cameroon, Cape Verde, Ghana, Guinea, Libya, Madagascar, Mali, Mauritania, Morocco, Mozambique, Nigeria, São Tomé y Príncipe, Seychelles, Tanzania, Uganda, West Sahara, Zambia, and Zimbabwe. In all, the medical professionals, teachers, and construction workers in Africa numbered in the tens of thousands. In an episode that marred this otherwise stellar history of internationalism, Cuba supported the despotic regime of Macías Nguema in Equatorial Guinea by sending it military instructors, doctors, and forestry workers in the period 1973–74.[66] Cuba's military mission to Ethiopia, after a coup deposed Haile Selassie in 1974, deployed 15,000 troops, second in size only to Angola. From the late 1970s through the mid-1980s, Ethiopia also received the second-largest number of aid workers. There they attended over a million patients during a year and a half.[67]

The Cuban medical mission to Algeria, after the country won its independence in 1962, set a precedent for many future missions. In 1979 when refugees from Western Sahara flocked to the southwestern Algerian town of Tindhouf, Cuba went to help them. Dr. González Polanco, part of a medical brigade of fourteen in that town, remembers that he did not get exactly what he hoped for when signing up for an international mission: "I said I'd go as long as it was in a place where I could drink coffee, where there weren't flies and where it wasn't too hot. But when I got there I found that there were lots of flies and heat, and no coffee. It was a sea of sand."[68]

As in so many other countries, local doctors would not travel to where they were most needed: the refugee camp thirty to forty kilometers from Tinfhouf. This meant that Cuban doctors were the only ones attending to the refugees.

Cuban medical assistance had to be more discreet in Latin America and the Caribbean, where the United States was eager to eliminate Cuban health brigades whenever possible. In 1970, Cuba provided disaster relief to Peru after the earthquake, later sending a construction brigade to help build six hospitals. Two years later, Jamaica elected Michael Manley as prime minister. Manley was friendly to the Cuban Revolution, and a brigade of fifty doctors went to Jamaica in 1979. With more than five hundred aid workers, Jamaica had the largest contingent in the Western Hemisphere. Edward Seaga defeated Manley in the elections of October 1980, and the new regime bent to Reagan's wishes, breaking diplomatic relations with Cuba and expelling virtually all aid workers by October 1981.[69]

Maurice Bishop's New Jewel Movement led Grenada's first successful revolution in March 1979, and by June of that year a Cuban medical team arrived on the island. The brigade had expanded to twenty health workers by 1982, which meant a 42 percent increase in the number of health professionals in the island and a 25 percent decrease in Grenada's infant mortality. The United States invaded Grenada in 1983, and the Cuban aid workers were expelled.[70]

In July 1979, the Sandinistas defeated the Somoza dictatorship in Nicaragua. Cuba soon deployed about two thousand aid workers there—mostly doctors and teachers. By 1984, 5,300 Cubans were working in health care in Nicaragua, which was receiving more medical aid than any other country in the hemisphere. In 1987, Cuban medical brigades in Nicaragua attended to some 856,000 patients. Though the U.S.-sponsored Contra murders exhausted the country, leading to the 1990 electoral defeat of the Sandinistas, Nicaragua did not experience the same blanket expulsion of Cuban medical workers as had happened in Jamaica and Grenada. The doctors were so popular among Nicaraguans that the new anti-Sandinista government allowed 167 to remain. During this time, small Cuban brigades also went to Bolivia, Colombia, Guyana, Mexico, Panama, Suriname, and St. Lucia.[71]

Two countries receiving Cuban aid were of particular interest. On April 26, 1986, a nuclear reactor at Chernobyl in Ukraine melted down, ultimately leading to an estimated 985,000 deaths and millions of sicknesses. Cuba flew in 25,000 victims for treatment, most of whom were children, with the first arriving in March 1990. The victims were not required to pay for their medical treatment, housing, or activities and Ukraine was only expected to cover transportation costs, which by 2015 it had not done. Laos is noteworthy because the two authors who cite the largest amount of official data indicate that Cuban doctors arrived there after 1975. Dr. Julio López provided me with his unpublished autobiography that includes his personal narrative as well as photographed newspaper clippings of his work in Laos beginning two years before 1973. This suggests that there could be earlier dates for other medical interventions and additional countries where Cuba provided health assistance that did not reach official data banks.

These extensive medical brigades stood in the shadow of Angola, where the number of Cuban aid workers reached at least 700 to 800 medical professionals at a time. Depending on the circumstances of the country, aid workers could stay for a few months or several years, could go by themselves or with Cuban troops, and might be enthusiastically welcomed throughout their stay or forced to leave by changing political winds. Medical workers were often the largest group of aid workers—in Ethiopia they were the majority.[72] It was not unusual for medical missions to be combined with related aid work, such as constructing hospitals in Peru.

As it was providing health care overseas, Cuba was also supplying medical education abroad, both by training students in Cuba and in their home countries. Between 1975 and 1991, over 70,000 aid workers went overseas. The 43,257 aid workers that Angola received was more than all other countries together. Teaching was often combined with health care; for example, Cuba established a medical faculty in Jimma, Ethiopia.[73] From 1975 to 1991, Cuba brought over 50,000 students from around the world to study in its schools, covering the complete cost of their education. Almost 20,000 students came from Africa alone in 1988. Within that group, the greatest numbers were from Angola (over 6,000) and Namibia (about 2,500). Many, such as Sophia Ndeitungo who survived the Cassinga Massacre, began in primary school and stayed until completing a Cuban university degree. By 1984, Cuba had trained students, at no cost, from seventy-five nations, virtually all from poor countries where medical education at no cost was unheard of.[74]

Dancing Barefoot on a Razor's Edge

In 1984, Soviet General Konstantin Kurochkin became obsessed with the idea of attacking Mavinga, where Savimbi had relocated UNITA's headquarters. He promised Angolan leaders that it would demolish UNITA psychologically. Cuba thought it would be a terrible mistake, since the FAPLA would have to go through an area controlled by UNITA and depend on a supply line that it could not possibly defend. From the Soviet vantage point, Cuba had not shown good judgment in applying the guerrilla strategy in Zaire, the Congo, and Bolivia. The Soviets persuaded the Angolans to change their view by offering visions of the war ending soon, and FAPLA began its advance in August 1985. The operation was based on the disastrous assumption that South Africa would not deploy its aircraft. When South African air support came—always publicly denied by the apartheid regime—the result was a total defeat for the FAPLA. A *Washington Times* journalist report seeing "an area of utter destruction where MPLA vehicles—caught grouped closely together—lay twisted and blackened in the scorching sun, the stench of dead and decaying bodies thick in the air as swarms of flies buzzed."[75] Angola lost nearly two thousand troops, and the UN Security Council condemned South Africa without applying sanctions. Observing that the air strikes had been decisive, Fidel proposed to the Soviets that they provide airplanes and train Cuban pilots to fly them. No approval came from Moscow.

In August 1986, UNITA attacked Cuito Cuanavale without South African air support and was defeated by FAPLA, which confirmed Fidel's analysis. In 1987, General Kurochkin persuaded the Angolans to repeat the attack on Mavinga. Again, every aspect of the campaign was a repeat performance: Cuba refused to participate; South Africa sent airplanes, while publicly denying its involvement, and the FAPLA troops were slaughtered.[76] Then something amazing happened.

Savimbi publicly claimed that "his forces, alone, had driven off the FAPLA troops, " and he bragged about UNITA's "great victory."[77] This enraged the South African soldiers (who saw their mates die during the attack), which led to an even more striking occurrence. Ignoring his government's insistence on secrecy, South African General Geldenhuys told the press on November 11, 1987 that his forces had won the battle. This sparked intense global repudiation of Pretoria's military intervention in Angola.

Was the time now ripe for Cuba to launch an all-out attack on South Africa's position? This decision had Fidel dancing on a razor's edge. The most delicate balancing act was with the Soviet Union. Without Soviet financing, Cuba could not carry out the war. Without its military supplies, Angola's FAPLA would be unable to fight. But repeated bungling of strategic decisions on the part of the Soviets threatened every aspect of the war. No less sensitive was Angola, which was looking less like the promising experience of Guinea-Bissau and more like the internal strife that drove Cuba to leave the Congo in 1965. Dos Santos's government suffered from corruption and had strayed from the ideals of Neto. Yet the MPLA government, whatever its failings, was vastly superior to the one that Savimbi would usher in. Also, a victory in Angola would strike a mortal blow to apartheid. But Cuba could not go forward without approval from dos Santos.

After Reagan had been elected and spouted the most war-mongering rhetoric of any president, Cuba saved its most powerful weapons for self-protection in the event of an invasion from the United States. As Cubans grew weary of a decade and a half of sacrifice in Angola, Fidel knew that being too cautious might mean missing an opportunity that would never repeat itself. However, moving too quickly could cause a defeat that would demoralize and exhaust the Cuban troops, doctors, and people at home. Another factor was the ebb and flow of anti-apartheid actions inside South Africa, which could tie up its government's troops.

When Fidel and Raúl met on November 15, 1987, they knew that the forces of apartheid could be sailing into a perfect storm of self-destruction. Conflicts between Savimbi and Geldenhuys had brought

South African support to a low point. At the same time, thousands of white soldiers had become unavailable for service in Angola, because they were needed in South Africa to suppress dissent. Meanwhile Reagan's embroilment in the Iran-Contra scandal left him too weak to attack. Fidel and Raúl agreed that the hour had arrived to send vastly more troops and arms to Angola, including Cuba's best airplanes, top pilots, and most sophisticated weapons. On December 11 and 12, the first Cuban boatload of heavy equipment reached Angola. Cuba's Jorge Risquet gained approval from the Angolans right after Ulises Rosales left from Havana to Moscow to present a *fait accompli* to the Soviets. When the chief of staff, Marshal Akhromeyev, heard that Cuba was already enacting its military plan, "he pressed down hard on the pencil and broke the point."[78]

Havana's military campaigns in Africa during the 1960s had given it experience in secretly moving men and arms across the Atlantic, which proved essential in this phase of the Angolan war. Though it might be doubtful that Fidel designed the entire family doctor program, there can be no doubt that he pored over every strategic and tactical aspect of the assault on South African positions, knowing that any mistake could cost thousands of lives. On March 23, 1988, FAPLA and Cuba defended the town of Cuito Cuanavale as it was attacked by South African and UNITA troops. Enough Cuban planes and pilots had arrived for them to score a victory in the air. At the same time Angolan troops drove back the ground attack. South African troops were demoralized as the battle signaled the beginning of the end of South Africa's adventures in Angola. Nelson Mandela observed that this key confrontation had "destroyed the myth of the invincibility of the white oppressor."[79] The incompetency of Soviet strategy had been exceeded by the blunders of UNITA and South Africa, confirming that the victor in politics and war is often the side making the fewest mistakes.

By August 1988, there were 55,000 Cuban troops equipped with the most modern weapons in Angola. Despite the clear defeat of apartheid forces, U.S. diplomats continued to tell their Soviet counterparts that South Africa would not leave Angola until all Cuban troops were gone. Fidel told the Soviet negotiator to "ask the Americans why has the army of the superior race been unable to take Cuito, which is defended by blacks & mulattoes from Angola and the Caribbean?"[80] Still wary that South Africa might launch a massive air attack from Namibia, Havana told Moscow that its troops would cross into that country if necessary. Getting wind of these plans was exhilarating for Namibian students, miners, and religious leaders, who realized that they were now part of a much greater military effort.

In the June 1988 negotiations, the South Africans insisted that all Cuban troops leave Angola, that Savimbi come to political power, and that Namibia become independent "in a manner acceptable to South Africa." Upon reading their demands, Fidel yelled, "This is a proposal written by idiots!" Cuban negotiator Risquet politely told them, "The South Africans must understand that they will not win at this table what they have failed to win on the battlefield." The apartheid negotiators represented a right-wing government chosen by white voters during elections of May 6, 1987. As they whined that an open acceptance of defeat would make it difficult for them to explain why they had been in Angola for so many years, they revealed that South African politicians had been telling voters that their troops were in Angola while denying the same to the international press. Knowing that a full invasion of Angola would be rebuffed internationally, result in thousands of casualties, and leave South Africa open to an internal black rebellion, the apartheid regime eventually ordered its commanders to leave. All South African troops withdrew from Angola by August 30, 1988.[81]

Even as their troops departed, South African leaders continued their antics. They had troops photographed with pretend smiles as articles claimed that South Africa ended the war on its own terms due to magnanimously deciding to stop the violence. No one was fooled. In November 1989, Namibian rebels were elected to office with 57 percent of the vote. In Angola's elections, dos Santos of the MPLA defeated Savimbi (49.8 percent to 40.1 percent). In April 1990, South African president Frederick de Klerk legalized the ANC and the South African Communist Party, while he freed Nelson Mandela, who was elected to head the country in April 1994.[82]

TABLE 5.2: Number of Cubans in Angola and Americans in Vietnam

	CUBA	UNITED STATES
Population in 1975	9,438,445	218,963,561
Soldiers in Angola/Vietnam	337,033	2,594,000
Number of Deaths	2,103	58,000

Source: Author.

The United States had a difficult time accepting its defeat in this proxy war. During negotiations that took place on October 6, 1988, U.S. diplomat Crocker bellowed that his government was not interested in "negotiations that were going nowhere." Cuban negotiator Carlos Aldana responded that Havana would not leave Angola prematurely, because "Ours are not defeated troops, unlike the U.S. troops in Viet Nam."[83]

Many of the parallels between the United States in Vietnam and Cuba in Angola were striking, and both foreign interventions had a profound effect on public consciousness.

Table 5.2 shows the population of the two countries in 1975 (the year that the United States left Vietnam and Cuba became involved in Angola), the number of troops from both countries and the number of deaths for each country. Examining these figures reveals that about 1 in 28 Cubans went to Angola and about 1 in 84 Americans was in Vietnam. Of Cubans who fought in Angola, 1 in every 160 died there, while of Americans who went to Vietnam, 1 in every 44.7 died. Thus, Cubans were three times more likely to go to Angola as Americans were to go to Vietnam, but, once at their destination, Americans were three and a half times more likely to die in Vietnam.

Aldana hit the nail on the head when pointing out the fundamental difference being that the United States suffered defeat while Cuba was victorious. This was partly because Cuba was defending an actual country from invasion while the division of Vietnam into "North" and "South" was a figment of the imaginations of French and Americans, which is to say that no foreign invasion occurred. It was no coincidence that Cuba treated Angola as a sovereign state (despite many differences) while U.S. politicians had as much respect for Vietnamese as a puppeteer has for his many toys.

Cubans left Angola knowing that, as a poor and small country, they had defeated rich South Africa, humiliated the mighty United States, and defied the Soviet Union. No one appreciated their support more than South Africans, who opened Freedom Park in Pretoria in 2007. Its Wall of Names recognized the more than two thousand Cubans who lost their lives in the Angolan war. Cuba is the only foreign country represented on the Wall.[84] As they were planning their departure, Fidel told Risquet, "What I regret is that when we withdraw the troops, we'll also have to withdraw the aid workers."[85] Knowing that they would have been viciously attacked by UNITA if they had stayed, Cuban doctors and other professionals left Angola in June 1991. The returning Cubans would be surprised by what the next decade would bring. Angola was once again left without the foreign medical help it so desperately needed. And hundreds of thousands of Cubans were jolted by what they confronted back home in 1991.

A TIME OF THE UNEXPECTED

B y the end of the 1980s, revolutionary Cuba had accomplished a great deal in the area of medicine. On the domestic front, this included:

- Expanding hospitals and clinics and cohering them into a unified health care system;
- Creating *policlínicos integrales* and overhauling them to become *policlínicos communitarios*;
- Developing the family doctor-and-nurse model and replicating it across the island;

On the international front, Cuba had:

- Integrated military and medical interventions in Africa during the 1960s:
- Massively expanded military and medical interventions in Angola;
- Integrated its medical internationalism with teaching, construction, forestry and other aid programs;
- Developed health education programs in many countries visited by medical brigades;

- Brought large numbers of students to Cuba for education, especially medical education.

It is highly unlikely that any other country in the world, especially a poor country, could have achieved so many monumental health care innovations as Cuba did between the 1959 revolution and 1991. The United States probably paid little attention to Cuba's medical feats, because it was so focused on military issues: the Bay of Pigs rout, its inability to detect Cuban troops in Africa in the 1960s, and South Africa's defeat in Angola, first in 1976 and later in 1988. Fidel Castro emerged as one of the world's most brilliant strategists of the Cold War epoch.

For those returning from Angola who had lived through an amputation with little to no anesthesia or whose memories of that war were visiting the grave of a relative or comrade, the reality of the African intervention may have been less than joyous. Another reality was also clear to Cuba—the United States had an intense desire to destroy the revolution in any way it could. Yet, the Angola campaign had given Cuba the knowledge, training, and experience to protect itself with troops and doctors, if a neighborhood-by-neighborhood defense were necessary. By 1991, its medical schools were full of professors who had visited numerous countries and had experience working in battlefield conditions, coping with the most serious combat wounds, and recognizing tropical diseases nonexistent in Cuba.

A New Disease Comes to the Island

During the Angolan wars, Cuba witnessed a disease it had never seen before. Throughout the 1980s, doctors began reporting a crippling series of symptoms described as AIDS. The disease was most rampant in sub-Saharan Africa, where more than a third of a million Cubans were going. In 1983, Cuba established a National AIDS Commission to create a prevention and treatment protocol. That year, Fidel asked the Instituto Pedro Kourí (which focuses on tropical diseases) to conduct research on controlling the epidemic. Cuba diagnosed its first AIDS case in 1985, and the first death came in 1986.[1]

In 1985, Cuba began testing those who had been abroad since 1981—including the large number of people who had been to Angola and other African countries—for HIV infection. Testing was expanded in 1986 to include other vulnerable groups such as blood donors, health workers, and pregnant women. By 1993, over twelve million tests had been completed, with results confirming a low number of seropositive people (under a thousand HIV cases), only 200 AIDS cases, and less than 125 new HIV cases annually.[2]

Cuba had passed a law in 1982 to create sanatoria where people could live if they had a highly infectious disease. When there was still little known about HIV/AIDS in 1986, Cuba took the emergency step of implementing a quarantine policy requiring those who had the HIV infection to live in sanatoria.[3] The policy sparked little to no concern inside Cuba, partly because most of those quarantined were military personnel returning from Africa. This group was accustomed to being assigned living quarters and aware of the need for nationwide public health measures. However, soon there was international outrage, especially from the United States, based on the claim that Cuba was violating human rights by targeting homosexuals through quarantine and registration. That this was politically motivated hypocrisy meant to fuel anti-Castro sentiment is confirmed by several factors that were typically ignored by critics:

1. Cuba often used quarantine to contain dengue fever and had registered patients with other contagious diseases such as leprosy.[4]
2. In the United States, sanatoria were used for tuberculosis patients during the late nineteenth and early twentieth centuries.
3. Children with poliomyelitis in the United States were often quarantined in their homes before the Salk vaccine was developed.[5]
4. At the same time Cuba was employing sanatoria, over a dozen states in the United States "brought AIDS within the scope of quarantine statutes."[6]
5. The claim that the Cuban government was targeting gay and

bisexual men is blatantly false, since those returning from Africa with AIDS were mainly heterosexual. The pattern of AIDS primarily affecting the homosexual community may apply to the United States and other countries, but it is not a global tendency. Cuba's initial pattern of HIV infection resembled that of African countries, where the disease primarily afflicts heterosexuals.[7]

6. As information on AIDS became more available, the quarantine was lifted. By 1989, sanatoria residents could come and go as they chose.

One might imagine that, after it became clear that the Cuban quarantine applied mainly to heterosexuals and was discontinued by 1989, then the attacks would stop. But that was not the case. The mass media continued to rant about the quarantine, some suggesting that it continued into the 1990s. Tim Anderson, in a study of HIV and AIDS in Cuba, points to how the charges were politically motivated:

> [C]riticisms must be seen in the broader context for economic "freedoms" in Cuba and in the context of US demands for the dismantling of Cuban socialism and for widespread privatization, including privatization of the public health system. By 1988, when homosexuals were still a minority of HIV-positive patients, they were beginning to be overrepresented. It was not until the 1990s—that is, after the quarantine had ended—that the Cuban pattern of HIV infection changed from the African pattern of affecting mainly heterosexuals to the Western pattern of affecting mainly homosexuals.[8]

THE COLLAPSE

After a number of Soviet bloc countries became independent and began moving toward market economies, the USSR collapsed on December 1, 1991. Following a meeting with U.S .Secretary of State James Baker, Mikhail Gorbachev announced that the USSR would remove its troops from Cuba and terminate its four- to five-billion-dollar annual subsidy. This was devastating for Cuba. It brought up memories of the resolution of the 1962 Missile Crisis, when the United States and the Soviet Union had also negotiated behind Cuba's back. The Cuban economy went into free fall: from 1989 to 1993 it shrunk approximately 45 percent, and imports dropped from $8.12 billion to $1.99 billion. Industry and transportation were hit hard by the drop in Russian oil imports from 13.3 million tons to 1.8 million tons during the same period.[9]

For decades, the Soviet Union had pressured Cuba to focus on producing sugar and nickel; now markets for both commodities declined since Eastern European countries could no longer purchase Cuban commodities at subsidized prices. Rubbing salt in the wound, the world price of sugar fell throughout the decade. Cuba's overall export earnings dropped 76.3 percent from 1989 to 1993. Productive industrial capacity had been at 85 percent in 1989, but the combined effect of the economic shocks knocked it down to 15 percent in 1993. Cuba's GDP, "which grew an average of 3.1% annually during 1963–89, declined 2.9% in 1990, 10.7% in 1991, 11.6% in 1992 and 14.9% in 1993, shrinking the economy to 65.2% of its 1989 size."[10] As Cubans witnessed this huge economic crisis taking shape, Fidel explained that they were entering a "Special Period in the Time of Peace." The Special Period would last from 1991 to 2000.

DISRUPTION OF HEALTH CARE

As the intensity of the crisis sank in, it raised the question of what would become of the medical projects that Cuba had devoted so much effort to in previous decades. The impacts on health were felt in three major areas: food intake, health care and services, and long-term health goals. Reduced ability to import food threatened the entire population. The average caloric intake went down 40 percent and the average protein intake decreased 42 percent. The effects were not uniform, however, since the government established nutritional priorities to protect children, pregnant women, and the elderly. Nutritional deficiencies hit adult men hardest, who lost an average of twenty pounds. Despite efforts to protect infants, the incidence of low-weight babies (weighing less than 2,500 grams at birth) rose from 7.6 percent in 1990 to 9 percent in 1993. This reversed progress Cuba had made during the 1980s.[11]

Intense shortages of running water, soap, and detergents disrupted daily hygiene. Electricity was often available for only an hour or two per day. Though the access of the typical Cuban to family doctors was not affected, pharmacy shelves were often bare. Shortages included medicines as basic as aspirin. One of the more dramatic problems was that low levels of vitamin B1 led to optic neuropathy, resulting in fifty to sixty thousand cases of temporary or permanent blindness. Among the drugs in short supply were those for treating HIV infection. (Paradoxically, the same sectors that falsely accused Cuba of discriminating against homosexuals with the 1985 quarantine, were now harming Cuba's gay community through an embargo affecting HIV medication.)[12]

The Special Period affected acute health care, most evidently through interference with ambulance service due to fuel shortages. Secondary and tertiary care likewise suffered, because Cuba could not rely on the Eastern bloc to supply medical equipment and replacement parts. According to MINSAP spokesperson Dr. Portillo, "There was a lowering of quality of care in the 1990s, when X-ray machines and laboratory diagnostic equipment were not always available." It was not easy to obtain replacement parts for radiology, mammogram, and cancer treatment equipment. Electricity blackouts made surgery risky, since power had to be supplied by generators.[13] Fortunately, many physicians had recently returned from Angola, where they had acquired experience with battlefield surgery.

In addition to creating problems with health care and services, the crisis affected Cuba's long-term goals in the areas of health care, health education, and international medicine. Julio López explained how the economic disruption interfered with his plans to transform childhood kidney treatment:

I was in Belize from 1989 through 1990 and went to Mérida [Mexico] to return to Cuba. I wanted to start an institute to focus on childhood kidney diseases, because I am one of the leading specialists in the area. It would have been called the Institute of Pediatric Nephrology. It was not possible to do so during that time in the Special Period, because we could not get lab equipment, because the country was moving backwards a bit. So kids with kidney problems had to be treated at a regular hospital.[14]

Faculty and students in all areas of the health professions had to cope with transportation in getting to and from schools and electrical outages when they got there. The shortages of medical equipment and spare parts also had a negative impact on education, and the embargo put an end to the purchase of medical textbooks from a Spanish publisher. International programs wound down as the country was unable to maintain its earlier level of work overseas. In Piero Gleijeses's words, "In the early 1990s Cuba withdrew its soldiers and its technical experts from Africa. Only fragments of the once massive aid program remained."[15]

STRANGLEHOLD FROM *EL NORTE*

The low point of the Special Period came during the years 1993 to 1995. Both the economic data and reports of the Cuban people show that this was when they experienced the most intense hardships. The United States did all it could to ratchet up the suffering in hopes that the island would implement a full market economy or descend into social chaos. The 1992 Torricelli Bill (Cuban "Democracy" Act) prohibited U.S. companies' foreign-based subsidiaries from trading with Cuba. The bill extended trade bans to medicines and food and prohibited ships that had visited Cuba from docking in U.S. ports for six months. Senator Robert Torricelli, who authored the bill, bragged that it was designed to "wreak havoc on the island."[16]

The Helms-Burton Act (Cuba "Liberty and Democratic Solidarity" Act) sought to dissuade non-U.S. companies from trading with Cuba. It also aimed to help Cuban-Americans to reclaim property expropriated decades earlier. The Cuban government held public events explaining that the law would allow expatriates "to seize private homes, public schools, union halls, day-care centers, sugar mills and other property." After initial hesitation, President Bill Clinton signed the act into law on March 12, 1996. U.S. pressure on Cuba continued into the next century as George W. Bush escalated the embargo and threatened the country militarily, while Secretary of State Colin Powell planned for the island's forced transition to capitalism.[17] Whatever the party or president in power, the U.S. government attempted to force Cuba into submission. Just as there had been bipartisan support for racist forces in southern Africa, so both Democrats and Republicans worked to break a country dedicated to improving universal health care at home and helping people abroad.

CUBA ADJUSTS

As the crisis began, Cuban planners proposed to inch toward a mixed economy under tight government control and thereby increase economic relations with other countries. Some of the most important legal modifications were:

1. Cuba legalized financial associations with foreign investors in 1992. Later, in 1996, restrictions on private foreign investment were relaxed to allow businesses to be 100 percent foreign-owned, with government approval and supervision. The main sectors affected were the "tourism, mining, energy, telecommunications and biotechnology industries, along with tobacco, rum, citrus and fishing."[18]
2. The U.S. dollar was legalized for day-to-day transactions in 1993, easing the ability of the 30 to 40 percent of Cubans with relatives abroad to spend money received from them.[19]
3. A new currency, the CUC (convertible peso) was created in 1994 to parallel the value of the U.S. dollar. The everyday Cuban currency is the peso, and it generally has an exchange rate of about 25:1 with the dollar or CUC. The circulation of CUCs makes it easier for visitors to spend in Cuba.[20]

4. Self-employment was permitted under government control in 1993 and expanded in 1995. This modification gave rise to the many tiny shops throughout the island and the small restaurants called *paladares* which Cubans often set up in their homes.

5. Most state farms became agricultural cooperatives, in which workers collectively own the products and divide money made from sales to the government or in markets. [21]

6. Farmers' markets and other markets were legalized in 1994, encouraging the sale of fresh produce and the existence of a huge variety of small shops.[22]

7. The government began to actively promote tourism.

The official endorsement of tourism had a huge effect on the economy and society. Anyone who has seen *The Godfather Part II* (1974) can understand why Cuban revolutionaries saw tourism as a source of depravity that had surrendered Cuban society and culture to the greed of imperialism. For this reason, the revolutionary government initially worked to reduce tourist activity, and when tourism became necessary Fidel called the policy changes "a pact with the devil." A necessary evil, tourism created jobs, a market for Cuban products, and a source of hard currency for imports. The total revenue from tourism jumped from $243 million in 1990 to $2 billion in 2002. The proportion of foreign revenue derived from tourism mushroomed from 4 percent in 1990 to 50 percent by 2005. In 1990, Cuba had 340,000 visitors. By 2003, the number had grown to almost two million and the tourist industry was employing 300,000 people.[23]

A new type of tourism allowed Cuba to use its medical experience and knowledge to financial advantage: health tourism. Foreigners could buy high-quality surgery plus a vacation for much less than it would cost at home. By 1996, health tourism was generating as much as $40 million annually. Both types of tourism compromised the ideals of the revolution. On the one hand, tourist sector workers were soon earning salaries many times higher than those in education or health, creating greater social inequality in the island. On the other hand, it soon became evident that foreigners were receiving higher quality medical care, a reality not entirely palatable, despite knowledge that income from medical tourism was plowed back into the Cuban economy.[24]

The documentary *The Power of Community: How Cuba Survived Peak Oil* (2006) portrays daily life of Cubans during the Special Period. Obtaining the most basic necessities was extremely difficult. For example, people often had to bring water to the upper floors of apartments with ropes and pulleys, and there could be three- to four-hour waits for buses, followed by idleness at work due to the absence of electricity or spare parts. To help people with transportation, government cars were required to pick up hitchhikers. Large numbers of Cubans had to begin riding bicycles, which was not easy in a culture without a history of bike-riding and whose new bikes were single-gear ones from China. Horses returned to many small towns as the primary means of transportation. Without pesticides or fertilizers, farming cooperatives learned organic farming methods and often plowed with oxen rather than tractors. Cuban research labs partnered with farming cooperatives to develop biological fertilizers and pesticides, not based on petrochemicals. Urban gardens popped up all over Cuban cities as fruits and vegetables became a larger part of the Cuban diet.[25]

The government asked "Cubans to sacrifice more by eating less, using less oil and petroleum products, working harder, and finding alternative ways to do things."[26] There was a massive proliferation of self-employment: not only work in *paladares* but also taxi-driving, repair services, and sale of personal hygiene products. With legalization of the dollar came "dollar stores" specializing in Western consumer articles. The policy of encouraging tourism meant that citizens could rent out empty rooms in their homes (a bit similar to bed-and-breakfasts) under strict government regulations. Taxes on these small businesses became a major source of government revenue, which was much needed to fund medical services.

RECOVERY FROM MEDICAL SHOCKS

Some public services in Cuba remained essentially unchanged, with no foreign ownership, no breakup of government entities, no reduction in domestic services, and no changes to allow self-employment. The most important of these were health care and education, which received revenues from taxes in those economic spheres where changes were made. Cuba's education and health care systems also benefited from decades of experience in massive literacy and vaccination campaigns. With an awareness of the gravity of the situation, every level of the medical system prepared to protect public health. Priority went to developing special mother-child diets. More maternity homes were created for women with high-risk pregnancies, with special attention given to the mothers' diets, while women with normal pregnancies were guaranteed access to workers' canteens. The Low Weight Birth Program was reevaluated for implementation at all levels of health care. The system for health records was also updated to ensure that problems would not be overlooked.[27]

The government made good on its promise to provide universal, free, and high-quality health care, regardless of the strain on the economy. Priority went to social spending, which included education and health care. In 1990, Cuba devoted a larger proportion of its governmental expenditures to social programs than did the United States, Australia, and Japan and twice as much as other Latin American countries. During the Special Period, Cuba's social spending increased, both in absolute terms and as a proportion of the economy.[28]

Even during the darkest days of the Special Period these government programs maintained the health system in three critical ways. First, no hospital was closed and even rural areas still had universal access to health care. Second, Cuba continued to prioritize medical education. There was only a slight decrease in the number of those admitted to health-related studies, which fell from 4,960 in the period 1988–89 to 4,846 in 1999–2000. Third, Cuba maintained its research institutes, working to develop new equipment, vaccines, and pharmaceuticals. Even though the government encouraged Cubans to obtain medicines from relatives living abroad, there was no evidence of a black market for drugs. One physician remarked during an interview that she had never seen illegal sales, and "If someone tries to do so, I will report it."[29]

Despite Cuba's success in maintaining its hospitals open, there were limitations on the care it could provide. Dr. Julio López remembered:

Hospitals were admitting more people and medications were being taken too often, when they needed to be conserved. So Cuba assigned more doctors to hospitals to ensure proper reductions in medication usage until more could be produced. Necessity created a greater development and education of a larger number of doctors to allow the shift to hospitals. Shortages were so severe that there were not even enough pens to write prescriptions. I went to South Africa in 1993. When I returned to Cuba in 1996 the situation was still bad, but people had accepted the reality of it and everything was much better organized. . . . During the Special Period, there was an increase in small weight births and premature births. Since there was less X-ray film, doctors had to rely more on their exam skills. If a doctor ordered too many X-rays, the medical director talked to the doctor about ordering fewer. It was the same way with lab work. If there were no clinical symptoms, the doctor was not supposed to order lab work. There were patterns of some doctors ordering too much.[30]

López told me that those ordering too many tests tended to be physicians with less experience. Those interviewed in 2003 remembered being pleased with primary care at *consultorios* and *policlínicos*. However, they recalled interruptions in procedures at both general hospitals and specialty hospitals, the latter being most affected by equipment shortages and breakdowns. Some visitors to Cuba reported seeing supplies such as syringes and gloves being washed for reuse. However, the health system was actually able to expand primary care, even if it cut back secondary and tertiary care services.[31]

The Global HIV Epidemic

One of the greatest medical challenges confronting Cuba during the Special Period was HIV/AIDS. The embargo exacerbated the shortage of drugs and increased their cost. Even more, the homophobia typical of Latin America was as rampant among medical professionals as it was for the rest of the population. Despite the false accusation that the quarantine was an anti-gay policy, the government put out its best efforts to fight HIV/AIDS. By the 1990s, when male homosexuals had become the largest group affected, school sex education programs, which began during grade five, recognized sexual diversity by describing homosexuality as a fact of life. There were also health campaigns, from the early 1990s forward, that encouraged the use of condoms, which could be obtained at no cost.[32]

As early as 1987, Cuba developed its own HIV diagnostic tests. Testing went forward for at-risk groups, including those with sexually transmitted diseases, prisoners, hospital inpatients, and pregnant women. From 1985 to 1993, 12 million HIV tests were carried out and, by 2003, at least 1.5 million tests were done each year. Zidovudine (AZD) was recommended for AIDS treatment in 1987. But such drugs were expensive, and Cuba was strapped for cash. Dr. Julio López told me that, due to the high cost of drugs, physicians treating patients during and after the sanatoria phase had to receive complete treatment authorization "at the highest levels." In 1996, Cuba provided antiretroviral (ART) drugs for children with AIDS and their mothers at a per person annual cost of $14,000. NGOs donated ART drugs for one hundred Cuban AIDS patients during the period 1998–2001.[33]

Cuban legislation ensured that HIV-positive patients could keep their jobs and 100 percent of their salaries after returning from treatment. Nevertheless, some Cuban employers attempted to get rid of HIV-positive people. In a survey of eighty HIV patients returning from treatment, 20 percent reported attempts to remove them from their jobs. One discouraged worker gave up his appeal and the other eleven with permanent jobs all kept them. But four with temporary contracts lost their positions.[34] Negative attitudes among health professionals were especially damaging. Dr. Gilberto Fleites, a cancer surgeon, recalled hearing Jorge Pérez declare at the National Cancer Conference that he was having a hard time finding surgeons to operate on AIDS patients. Fleites and a friend volunteered to help. This led to an important project:

> We started collaborating with the Pedro Kourí Institute Hospital, the tropical medicine hospital, which is the hospital for infectious diseases such as AIDS, malaria, and tuberculosis. We began collaborating and defending the rights of these patients to be treated the same as every patient—because no physician wanted to touch an AIDS patient. . . . They are afraid of being infected by operating on an AIDS patient. There is also discrimination, because there are many macho physicians. . . . Those prejudices still exist.[35]

Since Fleites had earned the ire of the government for his open opposition to the Family Doctor/Nurse Program, he worried that the heads of MINSAP might oppose his working in an AIDS treatment program. He encountered some resistance, but Pérez defended him, saying:

> Fleites, I don't care about [whether you are] white, black, gay or hetero, pro-Fidel or the biggest enemy of Fidel. I simply care that you are a good surgeon, that you are good with patients and that you put health and caring for patients above anything else.[36]

Willing to work with AIDS patients, Fleites managed to mount an operating room in the Pedro Kouri Institute Hospital and received money from the Global Fund for AIDS. Despite the treatment program he developed, a perfect storm of AIDS infection appeared to be brewing in Cuba. The HIV infection rate for the Caribbean region was second only to southern Africa. The embargo simultaneously reduced the availability of drugs, made existing pharmaceuticals outrageously expensive, and disrupted the financial infrastructures used for making drug purchases. Additionally, Cuba had long had open attitudes toward sex, with many adults having multiple relationships. To compound the problem of sexual contacts, tourism brought an increase in prostitution. If these concurrent factors were not enough, homophobic attitudes (which persisted among employers and health professionals) might have discouraged people from seeking testing and treatment. The key question was: Would the Cuban medical system be able to face these converging threats, or would it succumb to a massive epidemic that would rival the effects of measles and chicken pox that had arrived with European invaders to the New World?

REBOUND

Early in the Special Period, rates of HIV/AIDS infection in Cuba were favorable in comparison to those of other countries. At that time, medical anthropologist Nancy Scheper-Hughes discovered that whereas in "France and Brazil thousands of people have been infected with HIV-contaminated blood and blood products; only nine Cubans have been infected through a blood transmission." Cuba and New York City have roughly the same population. Yet when Cuba had only two hundred AIDS cases and one childhood death, New York City had as many as forty-three thousand AIDS cases.[37] This was in the early 1990s, when it was far more likely that southern Africa had been visited by Cubans than by New Yorkers. The issue was, as Cuba transitioned to having predominantly homosexual AIDS patients, could its research, health care, and social programs continue to keep the infection rate low?

As the Special Period wore on, the government intensified educational campaigns for schools, health care workers, and every other portion of the population. Tim Anderson describes two such efforts:

The educational text *Living with HIV* covers clinical information, HIV and the social environment, information on mutual

help, nutrition and hygiene, sexuality, and some legal consider-
ations. It explains the details of drug therapy, the development
of mutual aid groups and self-help strategies, and the rights and
duties of HIV-positive persons, as well as work, social security, health and confidentiality law. A second booklet, *Living
Together with HIV*, is designed for the families of HIV-positive
individuals.[38]

In 2003, Dr. Byron Barksdale pointed out how Cuba's six-week program for AIDS patients was "certainly a longer time than is given to
people in the United States who receive such a diagnosis. They may
get about five minutes of education." Along with mass education, the
government carried out nationwide tracking of HIV cases and their
partners, which appears to have been successful in detecting 75 to 87
percent of HIV infections.[39] Another factor was that, in contrast to
other countries, where one agency may have little to no idea of what
another agency is doing, Cuba carefully coordinates the work of government agencies, school, health care facilities, and communities—a
practice it calls "intersectional coordination."

Cuban research institutes went into high gear in the Special Period,
looking for generic drugs to treat AIDS infection. Its biomedicine
industry had produced zidovudine by 1998 and nine additional
medications by 2001. During that year, Cuba was able to provide all
of its HIV-positive patients with a comprehensive cocktail of ART
drugs, without charge. By impeding secondary infections, these
drugs caused the death rate from HIV/AIDS to plummet. In 2001,
the United States only provided 70 percent ART coverage, but Cuba
had attained 100 percent coverage.[40] The incidence of AIDS did rise
during the Special Period, but not as rapidly as it did elsewhere. When
the HIV infection rate in Cuba was 0.5 percent, it was 2.3 percent in
the Caribbean region and 9.0 percent in southern Africa. In 1997,
Chandler Burr wrote in *The Lancet* that Cuba had "the most successful national AIDS programme in the world."[41]

At the dawn of the new millennium, the comparative success
of Cuba's efforts became even more evident. During the period

1991–2006, Cuba had a total of 1,300 AIDS-related deaths; by contrast, the less populous Dominican Republic had 6,000 to 7,000 deaths annually. In 2002, neighboring Haiti was experiencing 30,000 AIDS deaths annually, and had 200,000 orphaned children. The United Nations echoed Burr's report in *The Lancet*, stating that Cuba's AIDS program was "among the most effective in the world."[42] By the end of the Special Period it was evident that continuing Western propaganda regarding the 1986–89 quarantine was to distract attention from the fact that Cuba had implemented a program to combat HIV/AIDS that was better than most countries', and, in particular, superior to U.S. efforts.

When three Cuban health professionals were asked what they thought were the reasons for the AIDS program's success, none of them felt that quarantine had helped. A typical response was that of a nurse-specialist who pointed to "the constant care given to the persons with HIV, and to their families; secondly, the united work of all the social and health organizations in this country, but above all it's the human effort." In effect, Cuban policy continually placed a strong emphasis on social support. The work Cuba did to overcome homophobia, even if incomplete, also played a role. In 2006, Fidel said, "Homosexuals were victims of discrimination. . . . I would like to think that discrimination against homosexuals is a problem that is being overcome."[43] Unfortunately, the combined effects of Fidel's speeches, the anti-discrimination laws, changes in school curricula, pamphlets by MINSAP, and the creation of the sex education center CENESEX by Mariela Castro were not enough to overcome anti-gay prejudice. In fact, the front line in the struggle against homophobia in Cuba—as in the United States and most other countries—is the often intense conversations between physicians, social service employees, employers, co-workers, neighbors, friends, and family members.

The anti-AIDS program was part of a larger, generally successful struggle to maintain health care during the Special Period. As years went by, the country not only recovered from medical setbacks of the early 1990s but even rebounded to a better level of care than existed before the Special Period. Between 1989 and 2003, Cuba saw

TABLE 6.1: Infant Mortality in Cuba and the United States, 1990–2017 (per 1,000 live births)

YEAR	CUBA	UNITED STATES
1990	10.5	9.4
1991	9.8	9.1
1992	9.2	8.8
1993	8.8	8.5
1994	8.5	8.2
1995	8.3	8.0
1996	8.1	7.7
1997	7.6	7.5
1998	7.1	7.3
1999	6.6	7.2
2000	6.3	7.1
2001	6.1	7.0
2002	6.0	6.9
2003	6.0	6.8
2004	5.8	6.9
2005	5.6	6.8
2006	5.4	6.7
2007	5.1	6.5
2008	5.0	6.5
2009	4.8	6.4
2010	4.6	6.2
2011	4.5	6.1
2012	4.5	6.1
2013	4.4	6.0
2014	4.3	5.9
2015	4.3	5.8
2016	4.2	5.7
2017	4.1	5.7

Source: World Health Organization, http://apps.who.int/gho/data/node.main.525?lang=en.

increases in maternity homes (86.5 percent), homes for the disabled (47.8 percent), elderly day-care facilities (107.8 percent), and research institutes (18.2 percent). The Family Doctor/Nurse Program, which covered only 46.9 percent of Cubans in 1990, expanded to 98.3 percent coverage by 1999 and 99.2 percent by 2003. There was also a rise in the number of health professionals to cope with the increased delivery of care, with the number of physicians increasing by 76 percent, dentists by 46 percent, nurses and nurses' aides by 16 percent, and technicians and assistants by 31 percent in the period 1990–2003. When adjusted for population growth of 5.6 percent these figures are equally impressive, as indicated by declines in the ratios of population to health care professionals. Between 1990 and 2003, the number of citizens per physician went down from 277 to 166; for dentists, the decline was 1,538 to 1,111; for nurses and nurses' aides, from 155 to 141; and for technicians and assistants, from 206 to 166.[44] Housing shortages during the Special Period meant that Cuba had to relax its policy of having family doctors and nurses live in the neighborhoods they served. By the 2000s, roughly 45 percent of physicians were family doctors, but only about half were able to live in the neighborhood where they worked. Nevertheless, accessibility remained excellent. Patients told Kamran Nayeri and Cándido López-Pardo that there was "no need for an appointment to see their family physician or to visit the attending physician at the polyclinic." When at the Vedado polyclinic they never saw more that four patients waiting and waits never lasted more than fifteen minutes.[45]

Even though Cuba had a problem of rising infant mortality during the first years of the revolution, it showed a continuous decline during the most difficult years of the Special Period. Table 6.1 shows how in 2000 the rate of infant mortality was 6.3 per 100,000 live births when the U.S. rate was 7.1 The gap between the countries continued to widen until, by 2017, Cuba's infant mortality was 4.1 compared to the United States' rate of 5.7. It is noteworthy that the first time infant mortality in Cuba fell below that of the United States was in 1998, toward the end of the Special Period, which points to the effectiveness of the many emergency measures implemented at that time.[46] Most impressive is the fact that Cuba's decreased mortality rates of women, infants, and children was not found in other Latin American and Caribbean countries at the time of the Special Period. The WHO's Millennium Development goals included lowering the 1990 under-five mortality rate by two-thirds by 2015. Cuba reached that goal by 2000.[47]

When I asked Dr. Julio López how it was possible to decrease infant mortality during the Special Period, he pointed to Cuba's ongoing medical advances and its physicians' capacity to adapt to crisis conditions:

Vaccination campaigns had been completed by then and were working. . . . There was special attention for high-risk infants. Popular education increased; there were changes in customs; medical treatment was improving; and doctors' application of what they had learned was improving. There was more attention given to sick kids, especially if they were less than one year old. There was an aggressive study of diarrhea-caused deaths. Earlier, it was thought they were due to bacterial infections but it was discovered that they were mostly viral and anti-bacteria medications were being overused. Then use of antibiotics was prohibited unless there was proof of bacterial infection.[48]

For an undernourished population, the starting point for improving health is increased food intake. Though the number of calories consumed per person decreased sharply during the middle years of the Special Period, by 2001 it had rebounded to 2916 calories per person, similar to the 1989 level. With help from its research institutes, vaccination campaigns and family doctors, infections and deaths from disease went down. Cuba's rate of tuberculosis was one of the lowest in the Americas. It vaccinated 98 percent of children under one against measles. By the end of the Special Period, it had eradicated measles, rubella, whooping cough, and parotisis (inflammation of one or both parotid glands, major salivary glands located on either side of the face).[49]

The campaign to control dengue hemorrhagic fever (DHF) during the years of the economic crisis illustrates how Cuba reconceptualized previous medical practices. During a 1981 outbreak of DHF, Cuba developed "active surveillance" techniques that included inspections, education, vector controllers (standing water and bromeliad plants), spraying, and "open hospitalization," which included "mobile field hospitals during the crisis with a liberal policy of admissions." Cuba also used "passive surveillance," which included testing potential cases. The country expanded this approach by adding new surveillance techniques when another dengue outbreak happened in 1997. Increased testing of hospital patients was combined with data from active surveillance to produce predictions concerning secondary infections related to death rates. These combined health policies were followed by reduced incidence of dengue and decreased mortality.[50]

Hospital care improved as Cuba began importing medical equipment from Germany, Brazil, and the Netherlands. The number of

TABLE 6.2: Life Expectancy in Cuba and the United States, 1960–2016

	1960	1970	1980	1990	2000	2010	2016
Female - Cuba	65.9	71.7	75.5	76.7	78.9	80.2	81.3
Female - U.S.	73.1	74.7	77.5	78.8	79.5	81.1	81.0
Male - Cuba	62.6	68.5	72.2	72.9	74.9	75.9	76.8
Male - U.S.	66.6	67.1	70.0	71.8	74.0	76.2	76.0
All - Cuba	64.2	70.0	73.8	74.7	76.9	78.0	79.0
All - U.S.	69.8	70.8	73.7	75.2	76.8	78.7	78.5

Source: https://www.worldlifeexpectancy.com/country-health-profile/cuba.

surgeries performed annually, which had fallen to a low point in 1995, began to climb back up.[51] A combination of maintaining critical funding for primary care and research along with developing new techniques meant that by the end of the Special Period Cuba had a life expectancy about the same as the United States. As Table 6.2 shows, the U.S. life expectancy for men was 74 years and 79.5 years for women in 2000. That same year Cuban life expectancy was 75 years for men and 79 years for women.[52]

As the new millennium began, Cuba had a number of significant achievements to boast of: it had adjusted to the lack of Soviet support; maintained its health system; weathered the HIV/AIDS epidemic; protected the care of mothers and infants; continued health education and training; increased the scope of the health services available for its citizens; matched the United States in life expectancy; and surpassed it in controlling infant mortality. The economic crisis had neither destroyed Cuba's ability to provide for itself nor undermined its people's health.

RENEWED MEDICAL MISSIONS AND ELAM

There was another dimension of health care that Cuba did not abandon during the 1990s: medical missions. In spite of the overall reduction of its international medical aid, Cuba went on supporting the victims of the 1986 Chernobyl accident throughout the Special Period. The nuclear power plant at Chernobyl, in Ukraine, melted down on April 26, 1986, when Cuba was the most heavily entangled in the Angolan wars. Cuban officials thought that the town of Tarará, ten miles east of Havana—where a polyclinic and midsized hospital were located, together with a *Pioneros* youth camp—would be a good spot for bringing patients from the nuclear accident. The year before the collapse of the USSR, in March 1990, the first group of roughly 25,000 patients arrived. They were mostly children, and the aid became known as the "Children of Chernobyl" program. The program employed four hundred Cubans, including as many as fifty doctors and eighty nurses, and persisted through the worst crisis years (1993–94), with Cuba covering the costs of medical care, meals, lodging, and activities. Whereas most countries assisting the Ukraine focused on slowing the spread of nuclear contamination, Cuba worked to provide treatment. The Chernobyl patients, many with cancer and hematological illnesses, stayed for an average of six months in Cuba, although those with the most serious illnesses sometimes spent years there. The last of the Chernobyl children returned home in 2013.[53]

Another focus of international aid effort during the Special Period was South Africa, where so many Cubans had died while opposing apartheid. The country needed help because numerous physicians had fled when the apartheid regime fell. Like many other countries, South Africa reimbursed Cuba for its medical services, realizing that Cuba provided the best medical care for impoverished people. Dr. Julio López described his own work there:

In 1993, Mandela was president of South Africa and asked Cuba for five hundred doctors. Cuba sent 150 right away and I went with the next group of two hundred and later a group of 125 to 130 went. I went to a hospital with 1,300 beds, where there were a total of nine doctors, in the entire northern province of Bophelong. I was coordinating efforts in the province and had Cuban doctors sign contracts when they arrived, including the time of the signature. That was hard because I did not have a watch. Once when I was on call a black South African woman had a miscarriage and I had not done a D&C [dilatation and curettage] for twenty-seven years. A nurse reminded me of the steps for doing it since, with only nine doctors, nurses often had to do D&Cs.[54]

More typical Special Period international missions were responses to two disasters in Nicaragua where Cuba sent medical brigades in 1991 (after flooding) and again in 1992 (following a volcanic eruption).

As effects of the demise of the Eastern bloc wore on, three patterns of international aid emerged. First, the major powers significantly decreased international aid, as they had virtually no competition for humanitarian gestures. Second, as Cuba began to recover by the mid-1990s and resumed aid programs, it focused much more on medical aid and less on other forms of assistance, such as construction and education. Third, though Cuba maintained aid programs in Africa, Asia, and the Pacific Islands, it was providing relatively more aid in Latin America and the Caribbean by the late 1990s.[55]

A decisive year for Cuba's medical missions was 1998, when Hurricane Mitch ravaged Central America. The total rainfall of 75 inches during 33 hours was accompanied by wind gusts over 200 mph and wave heights of 44 feet. Ten percent of Central Americans—three million people—were left homeless because of the floods, mudslides, and destruction of infrastructure. The most common international response was to offer loans, which implied debts for countries that were already poor. In contrast, Cuba sent supplies and promised to send two thousand emergency medical staff. Of Cuba's 21,000 medical students, 14,800 volunteered to help. Cuban teams remained in Central America for years, unlike those from other countries, which tended to remain only a few weeks. Mitch hit Guatemala hard, leaving 268 dead, 106,000 displaced, 6,000 homes destroyed, and 48 rural health stations damaged. Cuban doctors arrived within seventy-two hours and immediately went to work in the most difficult areas, in jungles and mountains, where many Central American doctors did not wish to go. Often the only means to get from one place to another was by donkey, in canoe, or on foot.[56]

Devastation was even worse in Honduras, where Mitch swept away entire villages and left 6,500 dead, 11,000 missing, 1.5 million people displaced, and 70 percent of crops destroyed. The next year, despite pressure from the Honduran Medical Association, the government permitted Cuban doctors to stay, because of their popularity among Hondurans, many of whom had never been treated by a physician in their lives. Haiti was also pounded by a hurricane in 1998 (Hurricane Georges) which killed over five hundred people and left hundreds of thousands homeless. In all of Haiti there were only two thousand physicians who, as in so many other poor countries, were concentrated in the capital. By contrast, Cuban medical teams quickly dispersed to 95 percent of Haiti's municipalities.[57] Cuba's response to the 1998 hurricanes formed the basis of a profound transformation in its medical internationalism. The first component of Cuba's global medical solidarity was sending doctors overseas, which began within a few years of the revolution and continued nonstop as crisis interventions. Second, as more doctors went overseas they found that they needed to train people in medical fields, including the occasional creation of a medical faculty. Third, simultaneous with the second component, was bringing students from abroad to study health professions in Cuba. The enormity of the 1998 hurricanes led Fidel to offer a thousand medical school scholarships to students from countries most damaged by Mitch. The consolidation of their education at a single location near Havana became the fourth cornerstone of Cuba's medical policy. The school would be called the Latin American School of Medical Sciences, but was soon changed to the Latin American School of Medicine (now known internationally by its Spanish acronym ELAM) to indicate its purpose of training students to become doctors.[58]

At ELAM's inauguration in November 1999, Fidel pointed out that there were 1,929 students from 18 countries. Most were from low-income families and many were children of parents who had been tortured under Latin American dictatorships. Cuba covered the cost of their tuition, textbooks, lodging, and meals. At ELAM, they were taught by professors who had all been on international aid missions. Students were expected to return to their countries and help the underserved. In the first graduating class, the average age was twenty-six and almost half the students were women. There were students from thirty-three indigenous groups, and 71.9 percent were from working-class or rural backgrounds; 84.6 percent of the students who were enrolled six years earlier graduated.[59] The education offered at ELAM, geared to promoting medical care for all, contrasted sharply with the global trend toward privatizing medical care, which compels service providers to respond to market forces and neglect rural areas. As its recruitment expanded beyond Latin America, one of ELAM's greatest assets became the interchange among thousands of students from around the world, all committed to providing medical care to those most needing it.

Not every government accepted medical assistance from ELAM graduates. Only seven years after Mitch, Hurricane Katrina pounded Florida, Alabama, Mississippi, and Louisiana (where it was the most violent) in August 2005. The governor of Louisiana put out a call for help due to the large number of people needing rescue and medical assistance and the insufficient number of medical personnel in the state. Fidel Castro assembled 1,586 medical volunteers with tons of medical supplies ready and waiting to make the relatively short trip from Havana to New Orleans. Nevertheless, George W. Bush turned a deaf ear to the repeated offers from Cuba, even as the death count mounted to 1,800. Undoubtedly, Bush's silence reflected the attitudes of many wealthy Americans who would prefer to see their poor countrymen suffer and die rather than admit that Cuba had a disaster response capability superior to that of the United States. As Cuban medical personnel waited patiently to go to New Orleans, they were officially named the Henry Reeve Brigade after the New Yorker who died fighting for Cuba in its First War of Independence from Spain. The Henry Reeve Brigade became a key part of Cuba's emergency response teams, which are prepared to react to hurricanes, floods, volcanoes, sanitary disasters, and/or chemical spills anywhere in the world.[60] At the end of the twentieth century, with one in three Cuban physicians working overseas, Fidel recognized that "as the Special Period draws to a close, medical services have become the most important part of our economy."[61] The U.S. embargo proved no more effective in destroying Cuba's morale than Hitler's Luftwaffe bombing of London during the Second World War was for undermining England. Indeed, the revolutionary rebound from the viciousness of the embargo showed that it had nudged Cuba toward what decades of Soviet tutelage failed to do: make the island more self-sufficient by diversifying its economy from a single export crop of sugar to one that included tourism and medical expertise as major sources of revenue.

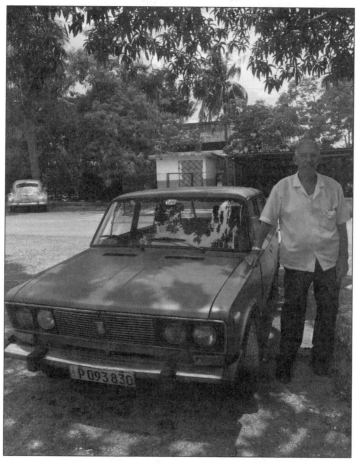

Cuban journalist Hedelberto López Blanch by his 1980 Russian car, Lada1600, June 27, 2019. Photo by Don Fitz.

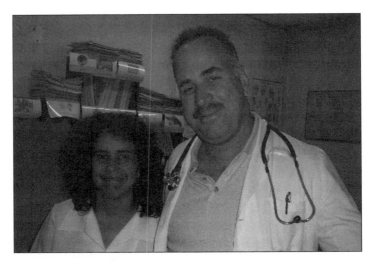

Dr. Alejandro Fadragas Fernández and nurse Maité Perdomo in Consultorio 5. Havana, December 30, 2009. Photo by Don Fitz.

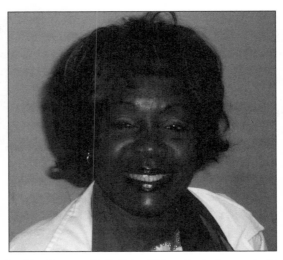

Teresa Frías, Vice Rector of Policlínico Universitario, has worked in Angola, Tanzania, Brazil, and Bolivia. Havana, December 30, 2009. Photo by Don Fitz.

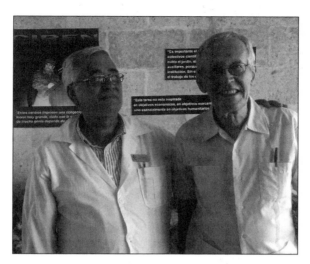

Dr. Carlos Suárez Monteagudo and Don Fitz in lobby of Centro Internacional de Restauración Neurológica with background photo of Fidel Castro at 1984 founding of the Center, June 27, 2019. Photo by Rebecca Fitz.

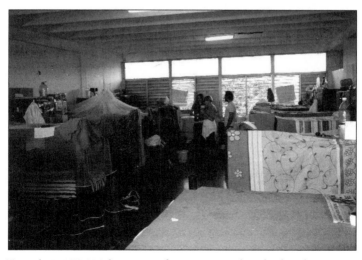

Typical 2009 ELAM dorm room for international medical students, 2009. Photo by Don Fitz.

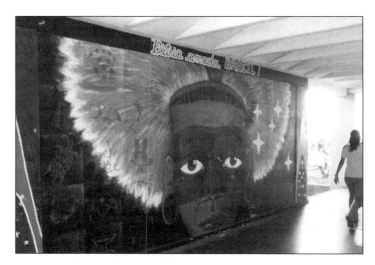

ELAM students from Brazil paint a wall, 2009. Photo by Don Fitz.

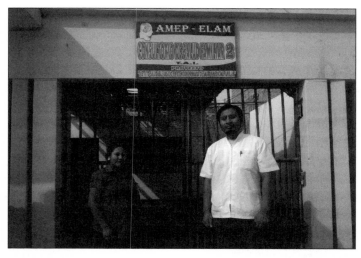

Drs. María Concepción Paredes Huacoto and Johnny Carrillo Prada, Peruvian doctors trained in Cuba, by Consultorio No. 2 in Pisco, Peru, December 2010. Photo by Don Fitz.

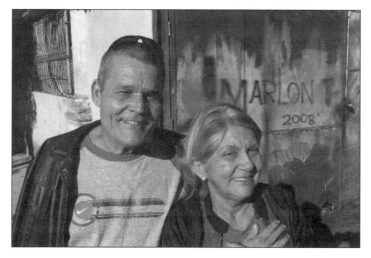

ELAM Professor Delfín Marrero and Deisy León Pérez by building for the Hermanos Zaís Committee for Defense of the Revolution, which she heads. Havana, December 30, 2009. Photo by Don Fitz.

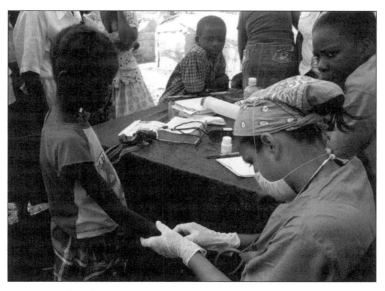

ELAM student does consultation with a Haitian patient, January 2010.

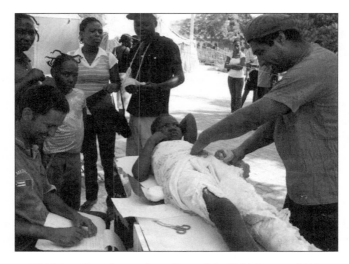

ELAM resident does orthopedic work in Haiti, January 2010.

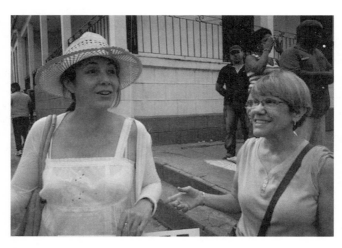

Mariela Castro and Barbara Chicherio, March Against Homophobia,
Cienfuegos, Cuba, May 17, 2012. Photo by Don Fitz.

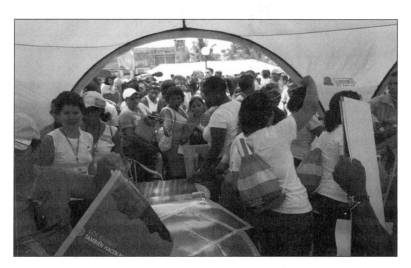

Getting gay rights posters after March Against Homophobia, Cienfuegos, Cuba, May 17, 2012. Photo by Don Fitz.

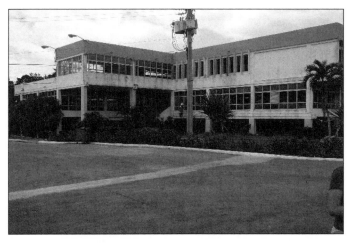

The ELAM building is a former naval academy west of Havana, 2009. Photo by Don Fitz.

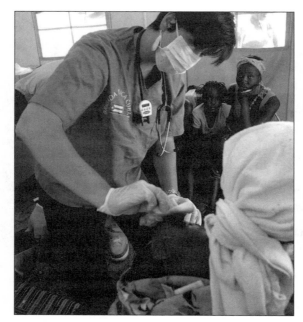

Joanna Souers attends to Haitian patient, January 2010.

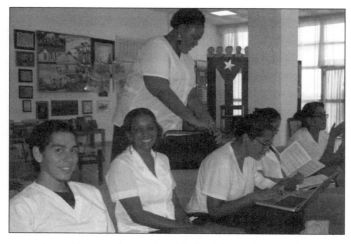

Several U.S. students at ELAM, 2009. Photo by Don Fitz.

— 7 —

ELAM: THE LATIN AMERICAN SCHOOL OF MEDICINE

We are one people who share a common history of struggle.
—CASSANDRA CUSACK CURBELO, SECOND-YEAR
ELAM STUDENT

A revolution can only be successful when the new generation takes over from the old. When thousands of students dedicated to helping others come together at a school that was built to allow them to fulfill their goals, the ground is fertile for those students to continue the struggle.

Students assume defining roles at the Latin American School of Medicine (*Escuela Latinoamericana de Medicina*, or ELAM), the twenty-year-old medical school in Santa Fe, Playa, a ninety-minute bus ride from Havana. With their educational costs covered by the Cuban government, students learn new social relationships in medical practice that they will use in their countries' underserved communities. This chapter details what I learned about ELAM during visits to Havana in 2009 and 2010.

INTERNATIONAL MEDICINE: A REVOLUTIONARY DREAM

In his article "The Cuban Revolutionary Doctor" Steve Brouwer describes a vision that Che Guevara had in 1960, the year after the Cuban Revolution. After observing that many graduating doctors did not want to serve in rural areas, Che imagined training *campesinos* to become doctors so they could hurry "immediately and with unreserved enthusiasm to help their brothers."[1] That year, Cuba sent medical teams to Chile to help after a major earthquake.[2] Cuba's first health contract resulted in its sending a medical brigade to Algeria in 1963.[3] In 1998, when Hurricanes Mitch and Georges devastated the Caribbean Islands and Central America, Cuba sent doctors and paramedics. In the aftermath of the hurricanes, Fidel Castro proposed expanding Cuba's new Comprehensive Health Program (*Programa Integral de Salud*) by creating ELAM, which began in 1999.

Fidel's ability to inspire changes cannot be overestimated. I met Exa Gonzalez, a sixth-year ELAM student, on a flight to Havana in December 2009. She had studied art and film in high school in Baja California, Mexico. As a teenager, she made two trips to Cuba with her parents, members of the Workers Party (Partido de Trabajo, PT). During her second trip, in 2001, Fidel described ELAM to a PT delegation, and inspired Exa to change her studies to medicine. She entered ELAM in 2002, when she was nineteen years old, and spent her first year in pre-med, studying biology, chemistry, and physics.[4]

Cuba's *Programa Integral de Salud* expanded dramatically in 2003, when the Venezuelan Medical Federation attempted to obstruct President Hugo Chávez's efforts to provide health care to underserved communities. Collaboration between Cuba and Venezuela resulted in the Inside the Community (*Barrio Adentro*) program, bringing ten thousand Cuban doctors to the country in less than a year.[5]

President George W. Bush refused Cuba's offer to help following Hurricane Katrina in 2005, which foreshadowed the attitude of the United States when Cuba began to provide assistance to Haiti in the wake of the 2010 earthquake. A friend told me that it must have been a publicity stunt by Castro, since he knew that Bush would not accept.

I replied that, given the breadth and depth of Cuban medical aid to countries in Latin America, the Caribbean, and Africa, it would have been an insult by Cuba to ignore the plight of a U.S. city near its shores. The high number of primary care doctors in Cuba makes it possible to move quickly after disasters like Katrina.

The U.S. media's slighting of Cuban medical solidarity continued through the 2010 earthquake in Haiti. As corporate news reports overemphasized U.S. aid, they seriously underreported Cuba's efforts, to the point of misidentifying a Cuban doctor as "Spanish."[6] In fact, ever since Hurricane Georges swept through the region in 1998, Cuba had assigned hundreds of doctors to neighboring Haiti. Additionally, Cuba has been training Haitian doctors since the doors of ELAM first opened in 1999. The only requirement is that, when they graduate, Haitians agree to return home to take the place of Cuban doctors (rather than defecting to plush jobs in the United States or Europe).

Cuba has already trained 550 Haitian doctors, and 567 Haitian students were enrolled in ELAM in 2010. As a result of Cuban efforts, Haiti saw a greater than 50 percent decrease in infant mortality, maternal mortality, and child mortality, and, between 1999 and 2007, an increase in life expectancy from fifty-four to sixty-one years of age. As Haitian president René Préval said, "You did not have to wait for an earthquake to help us."[7]

During the first three days after the earthquake, Cuban doctors provided more medical care than any other country. In addition to ELAM graduates already in Haiti, 184 Haitian students from ELAM (along with U.S. ELAM graduates) came to help, and Cuba soon had more than 1,500 medical personnel in Haiti.[8] This compared to 550 medical personnel from the United States at the same time. And, while the U.S.-based personnel had treated 871 patients, Cuban-trained staff had treated 227,143. Of course, Haiti was out of the headlines after a few weeks, and most non-military Americans departed. But, just as they were present before the disaster, Cubans stayed afterward, not just to treat patients but also to continue to build a new health care system.

Haiti is merely one recent example of Cuba's impressive international medical work. According to ELAM's website, there are 52,000

Cuban medical workers offering their services in ninety-two countries.[9] This means that Cuba has more doctors working overseas than
either the World Health Organization or the combined efforts of the
G-8 nations. Thus, "by 2008, Cuban medical staff were caring for over
70 million people in the world." Additionally, almost two million
people outside of Cuba owe their "lives to the availability of Cuban
medical services."[10] The spirit of international solidarity is at the core
of the teaching curriculum at ELAM. As its website announces: "The
work that ELAM graduates carry out today in all countries of the
world constitutes an example of internationalism and human solidarity. It is a symbol of love for life and social justice that is without
precedent in history."[11]

Student Health Brigades

After the third class graduation at ELAM, the Student Congress proposed creating the opportunity to work on specific projects during
summer vacation months. The faculty approved, and students began
designing projects designated as Student Health Brigades (*Brigadas
Estudiantiles por la Salud,* or BES) that would take them to clinics
in impoverished urban and rural communities of South and Central
America as well as throughout the rest of the world, including the
United States.

The Yaa Asantewaa Brigade (YAB), whose key organizers include
Omavi Bailey and Ketia Brown, illustrates how BES projects function.[12] YAB is the group that will carry out the "African Medical
Corp—Ghana Project." It was designed by the Organization of African
Doctors (OAD), a group of African and African-American medical
students. Founded in 2009 on the ELAM campus, OAD adopted the
mission of developing "programs, projects and institutions with the
objective of producing an organized, politically conscious and socially
responsible medical body able to meet the needs of African people
suffering from health-related issues throughout the African world.
OAD is composed of 160 students, interns, and residents trained in
Cuba currently representing over thirty-five countries."[13]

Currently, the "brain drain" of African doctors getting jobs in Europe or the United States leaves Ghana with just one doctor for every 45,000 residents. Similarly, there are more Ethiopian doctors in Chicago than in Ethiopia.[14] OAD aims to confront this problem head on by strengthening the directive at ELAM that African (and all other) medical students return to serve impoverished communities in their homelands.

The 2010 phase of the Ghana Proposal began with ELAM students traveling to Ghana to meet with Cuban-trained doctors already there. In the communities they visit, ELAM students intend to

1. Perform an assessment of the sources of health care that residents already have;
2. Establish groups of medical students who do physical exams and learn Ghanaian traditional medicine; and
3. Hold community meetings to strengthen ties with Ghanaian residents by finding out what health care they want.

Depending on the results, YAB hopes to create an internship so that sixth-year ELAM students can complete their medical training in Ghana. ELAM students in Ghana will have experiences that differ vastly from those of medical students in the United States. Unlike the overdeveloped countries, where the major causes of death are "lifestyle diseases" such as strokes and heart attacks, the principal causes of death in Ghana are preventable infectious diseases.[15] It is no accident that YAB aims to look at Ghanaian access to services, beliefs about health care, and desires for change, rather than jumping in to provide predetermined services that may not fit the life of an African village. Training at ELAM places heavy emphasis on the evolving social context of medicine, a model that applies particularly well to tight-knit communities.

Even though traditional and natural medicine are often ridiculed in the West, they remain the primary mode of prevention and treatment for 85 percent of African people.[16] Thus, the Cuban model of Comprehensive General Medicine (*Medicina General Integral,* or

MGI), which approaches health care holistically, considering its biological, psychological, cultural, and spiritual components, MGI prepares students to behave as doctors-as-listeners as much as doctors-as-teachers.[17]

GROWTH OF ELAM

The ability of Cuban-trained doctors to listen to people and work with them, rather than impose a Western model on them, is one factor that increases the eagerness of countries to send students to ELAM. Progressives in the United States who yearn for health care systems like those in Canada and Western Europe seem unaware of the tremendous prestige that Cuban-style medicine holds for impoverished countries. As Linda Whiteford and Laurence Branch observe, the Cuban health care system proves that "expensive medical technology is not necessary for effective community-based preventive care," having "eradicated polio, controlled malaria and dengue, and reduced child and maternal mortality rates to equal or lower than those of much richer and more developed countries like the United States."[18] ELAM offers the hope that other countries can accomplish similar goals. A six-year program, it graduated its first class in 2005. By 2007, ELAM had students from twenty-seven countries.[19] By 2008, the number of countries with students at ELAM had grown to forty.[20]

The ELAM Director of International Relations told me of how the school was expanding to campuses throughout Cuba. As of April 2010, the campuses totaled 21,018 students, from a hundred countries. Virtually all of Latin America is represented in ELAM. Even Colombia, with its notorious right-wing government, has 385 students. Students come from thirty-six African countries, plus many from the Middle East, Asia, the Pacific Islands, and the Caribbean.[21]

When I asked the Secretary-General of the ELAM Project if there were students from England and Australia, she said, "No, developed countries usually provide medical care and ELAM is designed to help poor countries."[22] This could be mistakenly interpreted as meaning that ELAM does not reach out to overdeveloped countries. However, if students are truly dedicated to working in underserved communities, they might be admitted if they apply through the Cuban embassy in their country. In fact, the 2010 matriculation table lists students from Germany, Canada, Israel, and Korea.

The internationalism of ELAM reflects the internationalism that runs throughout Cuban medicine. On the one hand, ELAM professors tell their students of having participated in relief efforts after disasters in Guatemala, Honduras, and Haiti. On the other hand, students also learn from other students about solidarity work in various African countries, Haiti, and Venezuela.

When students do rotations at neighborhood *consultorios* (doctors' offices) or community polyclinics, they work with medical staff having global experience. While visiting Havana's *Policlínico Universitario*, I learned from its vice rector, Teresa Frías, that she had worked in Angola, Tanzania, Brazil, and Bolivia. As her co-worker, also named Teresa, provided a tour of the polyclinic, she mentioned that she had worked in Ghana, Venezuela, and Brazil.

Any gathering of medical staff in Cuba is likely to include people who offer stories from distant parts of the world. "Internationalism" is not merely a slogan or ideology in Cuban medicine; it is a core component of a medical culture that permeates the country's way of teaching and practicing medicine.

Doctors as Teachers

Like many ELAM students, Ivan Angulo Torres of Lima, Peru, would have found going to medical school impossible. The costs were prohibitive and only one hundred students per year enter medical school in Lima. When he first heard of ELAM in 2002, Ivan was studying hotel administration. Two years later, he was in Havana. Four of his relatives attended his July 2010 graduation as the first doctor in his family.[23]

The course of study at ELAM differs somewhat, depending on whether students have sufficient pre-med background in biology, chemistry, and physics; whether they are from Cuba, Latin America, or a non-Latin culture; and whether they are fluent in Spanish. Rather than starting his school year in September, Ivan began his studies in March 2004, because he needed to first prepare with a half-year of science courses.

His first two years of medical school included basic classroom subjects such as anatomy, physiology, histology, biochemistry, genetics, organ systems, psychology, pathology, and the Cuban medical model, with its emphasis on public health. Ivan had contact with a neighborhood *consultorio* his first year and learned how to give physical exams his second year. During his third year, he began working with hospitalized patients as a practicum from 8:00 to 10:00 in the morning. He made rounds with doctors from 10:00 a.m. to 1:00 p.m., and took courses such as symptomatology, internal medicine, X-rays, and English in the afternoon.

His fourth and fifth years saw extensive training in the Cuban MGI model of medicine, which emphasizes people as bio-psycho-social beings, whose life context must be understood in order to treat them. The MGI model trains doctors how to teach patients to care for themselves, largely by changing the social context of their lives, including their communities. During those two years, Ivan studied public health and did two-month hospital rotations in areas such as MGI, ear/nose/throat, ophthalmology, obstetrics/gynecology, pediatrics, surgery, orthopedics, urology, dermatology, and psychiatry. During his sixth year as an intern, he was responsible for patients in a *consultorio* every day and for polyclinic patients one day per week. He also completed all his major rotations begun during his third through sixth years.

From the beginning of their training, ELAM students learn that the essence of public health is the neighborhood clinic, or *consultorio*. The medical system aims to deal with 80 percent of health problems in the *consultorio*, each of which serves about 150 families.[24] The *consultorio* is often described as a neighborhood doctor's office, with patients seen on the first floor, the doctor living on the second floor, and the nurse living on the third floor. This is the ideal Cuban model, but it does not capture the variety of forms actually employed or the close connection between medical students and the *consultorio*.

In December 2009, Dr. Alejandro Fadragas Fernández and nurse Maité Perdomo showed me their *consultorio*, which serves about five hundred families and 1,800 patients, making it larger than is typical in Cuba.[25] On the wall was a poster listing the "teaching staff" of two doctors, four nurses, two first-year ELAM or Cuban students, one fourth-year student, one fifth-year student, and an intern. The poster tells us many things. First, medical students are integrated into neighborhood health care, beginning with their first year of medical school. Second, Cuban residents are accustomed to international students being part of their treatment. Third, since there may be multiple doctors and nurses working at a *consultorio*, they do not all live in the same building. They live in the neighborhood or close to it, and the degree of integration into the community is complex. Fourth, medical teaching is not limited to ELAM but is integrated throughout the practice of neighborhood medicine in Cuba—doctors expect to help train medical students as part of their practice. This is so much the case that medical students often use the words *profesor* and *médico* (doctor) interchangeably.

THE MEANING OF ELAM FOR ELAM STUDENTS

Why do students from across the world come to ELAM? For Exa Gonzalez of Mexico, a speech by Fidel Castro changed her life. For Ketia Brown from California, ELAM's unique blend of traditional medicine with modern practice caught her eye.[26] For Cuban-American Cassandra Cusack Curbelo, a second-year student, it was an opportunity to share the dream of helping others by returning to the land where her grandparents had been revolutionaries.[27] But for many, it is a combination of being able to afford to go to medical school and participate in a vision. Ivan Angulo was not the only student who could never have afforded a traditional medical school.

Anmnol Colindres of El Paraíso, Honduras, had long wanted to be a doctor, but his father, who had been a forestry worker until the coup of June 28, 2009, could not afford to pay his way.[28] Amanda Louis, from the Caribbean island of St. Lucia, feels that she has an opportunity at ELAM that she never would have had, due to the low earnings of her father, a taxi driver, and her mother, a street vendor.[29] Dennis Pratt, originally from Sierra Leone, before his family moved to Jonesboro, Georgia, did not want to spend years paying medical school loans and immediately applied when he learned of ELAM.[30]

Like other students from the Pacific island nation of Tuvalu, Jonalisa Livi Tapumanaia is excited that ELAM will make it possible to put a doctor on each of the ten major islands of her home country, which is suffering from rising waters due to global warming. Her government can pay for only one return visit every three years; her father, who runs a gas station, and her mother, who works in an island court, cannot cover the cost.[31] It is also costly for Lorine Auma to visit her family in Kenya. She will see them only once during her six years of study. Her father, an accountant, and her mother, who sometimes works as a printer, could not afford Kenyan medical school, which is expensive.[32] Keitumetse Joyce Letsiela reported that there is no medical school in her native Lesotho, and her mother, a teacher, did not have funds to send her to an expensive medical school in neighboring South Africa.[33]

Clearly, a huge number, probably a majority, of ELAM students could not attend medical school were it not for its free tuition. One part of their education is learning that improving medical care in Cuba has meant focusing on preventive family care. Medical practice in the United States is so overspecialized that only 11 percent of doctors are family physicians. In contrast, almost two-thirds of Cuban doctors practice family medicine. While the ratio of family physicians per population is about 1:3,200 in the United States, it is about 1:600 in Cuba, the highest such ratio in the world.[34]

Many ELAM students I spoke with intend to practice family medicine. But several others feel that they should continue their studies after ELAM to be able to offer affordable specialist services in their countries. Ivan Angulo from Peru plans to specialize in orthopedics. Dennis Pratt hopes to practice pediatrics and internal medicine in

Sierra Leone. Ivan Gomes de Assis would like to practice orthopedics in Brazil.[35] Walter Titz, also from Brazil, would like to practice general medicine for a few years and then study psychiatry.[36]

Amanda Louis reports that her Caribbean home of St. Lucia has only one oncologist and one ear, nose, and throat doctor, but feels there are enough general practitioners and ob/gyn doctors. She would like to specialize in nephrology (kidney) disorders. Yell Eric thinks that there are many general practitioners in his African island country of São Tomé and Príncipe and is not sure if he wants to specialize or not.[37] When Lorine Auma returns to Kenya, she would like to focus on orthopedics or psychiatry. Perhaps most typical of the ELAM students I spoke with is Joyce Letsiela who is devoted to helping underserved communities in Lesotho and feels that there is a serious shortage of both general practitioners and specialists there.

CHALLENGES

Although ELAM has five hundred positions allotted for U.S. students, only 117 were filled as of April 2010. The Interreligious Foundation for Community Organization (IFCO), which screens U.S. applicants to ELAM, strongly encourages low-income people of color to apply. But the fundamental requirement is that students demonstrate a commitment to working in distressed communities.[38]

Many young people from the United States who think about going to ELAM find ways to contact U.S. students already there. An even better route is to contact IFCO and consider visiting the school. While on campus, it is easy to talk to U.S. students already there, as well as students from other countries who speak English.

A person's opinion of the quality of a medical school can be influenced by:

- *Physical appearance.* Compared to the luxury of U.S. medical schools, ELAM falls short. Running water is available only at certain hours, and toilets have to be flushed with a bucket. Cuba often has to sacrifice superficialities in order to ensure that everyone has necessities.

- *Quality of training.* Although ELAM provides books in Spanish, other books may be difficult to get. U.S. schools provide training geared directly to U.S. medical board exams, but ELAM students get more hands-on experience earlier.
- *Dedication to creating a new medicine.* It is in this dimension that ELAM surpasses every other medical school in the world. This should be the reason that students apply.

The evening before I departed from Havana, I had an extensive conversation about the ELAM experience with my daughter, Rebecca Fitz, then a third-year student, and her partner, Ivan Angulo, who had just finished his sixth year.[39] They detailed many things that ELAM provides at no cost: (1) classes and textbooks; (2) dorm rooms; (3) meals (three per day); (4) medical services, including emergency and elective surgery (many ELAM students receive corrective procedures such as eye surgery and braces); (5) items such as two student uniforms, stethoscope, blood pressure cuff, mosquito net, shoes, socks, sheets, blanket, winter coat, and silverware; (6) rations, including soap, toilet paper, laundry detergent, toothpaste, deodorant, and school supplies; and (7) a stipend of one hundred pesos per month. (For reference, an ice cream on campus costs one peso, while a beer costs about ten pesos; so students could chill out from studying by having a beer every three days.)

Conversely, ELAM presents challenges to students accustomed to life in the United States. The first requirement for acceptance is being able to document a history of commitment to social justice. ELAM does not exist to give people a free ride through medical school. Students are expected to show that they will give as much to their communities as ELAM gives them.

Though ELAM covers basic expenses while attending school, students must obtain their own transportation to and from Cuba. This is not an issue for most U.S. students, although they may not have funds to return home during the summer. IFCO encourages U.S. students to complete college-level courses in biology, chemistry, and physics prior to attending ELAM, so that they can concentrate on learning

Spanish after arriving. Students from most other countries can begin medical school immediately after graduating high school, and can take any needed science courses during an additional first year of pre-med.

Students must be able to live in a land without excess luxury. Most do not find this too difficult, since they are aware that Cuba maintains a life expectancy equal to the United States by devoting its resources to making sure everyone has what is necessary. The U.S. economic embargo ensures that there is not a great deal more. Students should be prepared to bathe from a bucket and live with hurricanes and without air conditioning. The cafeteria serves institutional food, which might be found lacking in variety. It is not unusual to experience difficulty in adjusting to the absence of things one is accustomed to, such as brownies, hot running water, or private personal space. There is a norm of being political, which is wonderful for many, but can be a surprise for some. For example, students are expected (but not required) to participate in activities of their country's delegation, and class discussions may include the role of their country in imperialism.

ELAM is designed for a majority of students who matriculate young, even at the age of sixteen. U.S. students, who tend to be older, may be surprised by requirements such as taking physical education courses or spending nights on campus Monday through Friday. Finally, a large majority of students come from countries that are eager to send them to ELAM to become Cuban-trained doctors. This is not the case with Brazil and the United States. In 2009, the Brazilian medical association, *Colégio Médico*, had policies distinct from the Lula government and did not recognize degrees from ELAM. U.S. students do not have this problem, but they must take the same exams as anyone does to receive a non-U.S. degree, and they need to study extensively for questions based on a U.S. rather than a Cuban medical model.

U.S. students cannot expect any support from the U.S. Interests Section, a substitute for an embassy in Cuba (a U.S. embassy does not exist, due to lack of diplomatic relations between the two countries). Though it is legal to travel to Cuba for educational purposes (such as medical school), the U.S. government employs more hostile restrictions on travel to Cuba than on almost any other country, and does nothing to support students at ELAM.

An Affirmation

Perhaps the extreme antagonism by the most violent country on the planet is an affirmation of the power of ELAM. The Cuban public health model seeks to understand medical problems by studying the wholeness and completeness of the human context of those problems. ELAM is central to Cuba's efforts to integrate its medical system with the needs of underserved people throughout the world. The Cuban model is based on a belief that the illnesses of humanity cannot be seriously addressed without addressing the society that creates the basis for those illnesses.

This model has attracted well over 20,000 international students. Cassandra Cusack Curbelo believes: "There is no experience like thousands coming together with the same idea of medicine. It feels like we are not separated into two continents, but we are one people who share a common history of struggle. This is what ELAM opens our eyes to." According to medical student Ketia Brown, "ELAM is the revolution realized. We must attempt to have a revolutionary project in a capitalist world." ELAM is such a project. It is a struggle for a new medical consciousness as a part of the struggle to improve global health.

— 8 —

THIRTEEN FACES OF ELAM

Cuba is doing more than any other country in the world to reverse medical "brain drain." A physician who leaves Sierra Leone for South Africa can earn twenty times as much money. Higher pay in English speaking countries of the Global North lures medical graduates from India (10.6 percent of doctors), Pakistan (11.7 percent), Sri Lanka (27.5 percent), and Jamaica (41.7 percent). Only fifty of six hundred doctors trained in Zambia remained there after independence in 1964.[1]

The Cuban alternative was founded in 1999 as ELAM (Latin American School of Medicine). With educational costs covered by Cuba, students prepare to return as doctors to underserved communities in their countries. The 21,000 medical students in Cuba receive much more than a free education—they are involved in building a new type of medicine. ELAM students learn the Cuban model of *Medicina General Integral* (MGI), which focuses on public health and primary care. MGI is based on a holistic approach to understanding health and disease that includes biology, sociology, economics, and politics. Cuban efforts to improve health care are based on creating a new medical awareness. This chapter, based on interviews I carried out in the period 2009–10, describes how ELAM affected the medical consciousness of thirteen of its students.

Exa Gonzalez

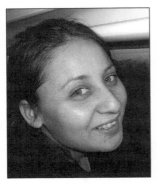

I met Exa Gonzalez over the Gulf of Mexico. She was sitting next to me on the airplane as I told her of the challenges I faced in visiting my daughter at ELAM due to U.S. travel restrictions. She replied, "I'm a sixth-year student there."

Exa is from the town of La Paz in Baja California, Mexico. Both of her parents had been active in the Partido de Trabajo (PT, Workers Party). In 2001, Exa and her parents went on two trips to Cuba with the Friendship between Cuba and Mexico group.

In high school, Exa was fascinated by art and took courses in film. But she was also interested in helping people and knew that Cuba had sent doctors to Central America for hurricane relief. On her second trip to Cuba, Fidel Castro described ELAM to her delegation. That changed her life. She decided that the best way to fulfill her childhood goal of helping people would be to become a doctor.

When Exa entered ELAM right after high school at age nineteen, she spent several months studying biology and chemistry in pre-med. Exa described her first year at ELAM as her "sad year," when she found herself in a culture very different from Mexico's and felt so alone she wanted to leave. With her mother's encouragement, she decided to stay. When we spoke, Exa was completing her final year.

Anmnol Colindres

As twenty-two-year-old Anmnol Conindres was waiting outside the Consultorio Médico No. 17-2 in Havana, he told me about his life in Honduras. His entire family had been affected by the June 2009 coup against President Mel Zelaya. His father had been a forestry worker. However, with the economic devastation following the coup, he lost his position and took lower-paying work as an agricultural director.

His twenty-year-old sister had to drop out of school before finishing because grants disappeared. Anmnol's seventeen-year-old brother had planned to study engineering in Venezuela, but those hopes were dashed when the new Honduran regime turned against Hugo Chávez.

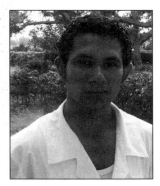

Anmnol had long wanted to be a doctor, but the costs were prohibitive. After studying to be a teacher, he learned of ELAM. According to Anmnol, Honduran students are selected for ELAM by a mixed system relying on exam scores, lottery selection, and recommendations. Due to his exam scores, Anmnol qualified to attend ELAM in 2006. Not having the resources to fly to Cuba, he had to work for a year.

Anmnol told me about the Honduras he would return to and the challenges of practicing medicine there. Under President Zelaya, Cuban-trained doctors had worked in Honduras, and ELAM graduates had opened a clinic offering medical care at no cost. However, the clinic was shut down after the coup, and thugs attacked the medical students and doctors.

Honduran doctors tend not to want to work in areas that have the greatest need. The Honduran Colegio Médico (analogous to the American Medical Association), which supported the coup, would like to privatize government-based medical care. There is a danger that it will not recognize Cuban-trained doctors. For that reason, it may be necessary for ELAM graduates to form their own medical association in Honduras. Since the country has too few medical specialists, Anmnol hoped to study cardiology in Spain before returning to work in poor areas of Honduras.

Ivan Gomes de Assis

Ivan Gomes was a twenty-three-year-old student from Salvador City in Brazil in his second year at ELAM. After finishing his studies, he initially taught mathematics in high school. His father was a lawyer

and Ivan's family had often helped people
receive medical care who were unable to
pay. When he was twenty, Ivan learned
of ELAM through the internet and was
impressed that the school did not turn
out wealthy doctors. He decided that
practicing medicine would be the best
way to help Brazil's poor.

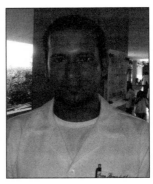

Brazilians are typically admitted to
ELAM through leftist parties, but Ivan
had no history with the left. Nevertheless, the Cuban embassy staff
endorsed him. After finishing medical school, Ivan wanted to study
orthopedics and practice in rural areas of Brazil where there are few
specialists.

Ivan found school at ELAM difficult, partly because the U.S. blockade made it hard to access the internet. He felt that ELAM is a great
school, but prefers to study independently and did not like receiving
a lower grade if he skipped classes.

Ivan was concerned about the way Brazilian doctors participate in a
grossly unequal and corrupt system. The Brazilian medical association
does not want doctors trained in Cuba to receive certification in Brazil.

WALTER TITZ

Walter, a twenty-three-year-old second-year student from São Paulo,

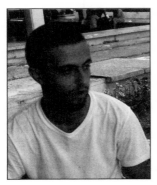

Brazil, dreamed of creating Cuban-
style community medicine in Brazil.
Walter had wanted to pursue a career in
medicine, but he went to the Catholic
University of Santos and studied journal-
ism. Since progressive parties in Brazil
recommend students, Walter realized
that becoming active in the Brazilian
Communist Party could be important.
He was also active in student groups

working in solidarity with the Landless Workers' Movement (MST).

Walter's father was a newspaper editor who had been active in the Workers Party, but due to disappointment with the Lula government, moved closer to the Brazilian Communist Party. Walter's mother, who worked in the judicial system, was not happy with her son leaving Brazil. Yet she supported Walter's work and was glad that he was attending ELAM.

Walter found an enormous difference between the political environment at ELAM and that of Brazil. Seeing how Cubans survive with very little—by having the necessities of life guaranteed—helped ELAM students envision how they could change their own countries. He told me how many Latinos came to ELAM thinking that there is no suffering in the United States, but they learned otherwise by talking with U.S. students. Through the experience, they also learned how the United States has destroyed lives. According to Walter, they were inspired by people from the United States who opposed U.S. imperialism.

Walter planned, after graduating, to return to his community to practice general medicine and then study psychiatry. Unfortunately, the rich, elitist Brazilian Colegio Médico did not recognize Cuban degrees. For this reason, Walter believed that Brazil needed to build a new medical system.

IVAN ANGULO TORRES

Ivan Angulo initially studied hotel administration in Lima, Peru. He told me it would have been crazy for him to even think of studying medicine. Only one hundred students per year were admitted to medical school in Lima, and even though his father was director of a secondary school, his family could not afford it.

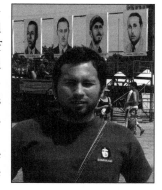

Ivan's father was a member of the Socialist Revolutionary Party (PSR), one of the left parties that can nominate young people to attend ELAM. Ivan became the first PSR-recommended student. At twenty-eight years of age, he had just completed ELAM's six-year program when I interviewed him. New Peruvian doctors from ELAM must work for a year in rural areas, where there is a shortage of all services, including medical care. He hoped to study orthopedics and practice either in Peru's jungles or in his family's home province. Ivan expected his Cuban degree to be treated in the same way as medical degrees from other countries.

Amanda Louis

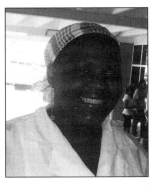

Amanda Louis, a first-year student from the small Caribbean island of St. Lucia, told me: "Cuba gives people like me an opportunity to study medicine that we would never have anywhere else." She was twenty-six when I interviewed her. Her father was a taxi driver and her mother a food vendor.

Amanda had graduated from high school in 2000, went to community college, and then taught integrated sciences and chemistry. She learned that the maximum age for admission to ELAM was twenty-five and applied right away. Though she had been a youth organizer in St. Lucia, her political and social work did not count toward admission. Rather, her school grades were the most important factor. Amanda was in the first class from St. Lucia to go to ELAM in Havana—previous classes had gone to other Cuban cities. Amanda hoped, after receiving her degree, to focus on kidney disorders. She told me that there were enough general practitioners in St. Lucia, but only one oncologist and one ear, nose and throat doctor in the nation of some 165,000 people. She said that students from St. Lucia would have no trouble with their medical degree being recognized in the country. Amanda would have to work for the government for five years to pay for her transportation and incidental funds. Though physicians in St. Lucia think that a degree from Cuba is not as good as other schools, Amanda thought it was better. "Here, they give us more hands-on work with patients at the *consultorios* and polyclinics."

Cassandra Cusack Curbelo

Of the ELAM students I spoke with, Cassandra Cusack was the only one from the United States who applied directly to the Cuban Interests Section in Washington, D.C., rather than through the Interreligious Foundation for Community Organization (IFCO). One of the few Cuban-Americans at ELAM, Cassandra was from Hialeah, near Miami, Florida. Her mother was born in Cuba and came to the United States with Cassandra's grandparents shortly after the 1959 revolution. The family migrated due to misinformation, and her grandparents soon felt tricked. They became strong supporters of the revolution.

Cassandra's grandmother had left school in Cuba after third grade, and her mother had to struggle hard to get her education. They both wanted to visit Cuba, which put them in conflict with most Cuban-Americans. Cassandra feels that the dictatorship that existed before the Cuban Revolution now exists in Miami. Nevertheless, she found that young people are far less hostile toward the Cuban government, despite the flood of horror stories.

It was sometime between her trips to Cuba in 1996 and 2006 that Cassandra decided to go to medical school. In the United States, she studied film and then social work. Before coming to ELAM, she was actively involved in antiwar coalitions, immigrant rights, animal rights, and anti-WTO efforts. She applied for admission to ELAM when she was approaching the age limit of thirty for U.S. students. Cassandra was thirty-one and finishing her first year in medical

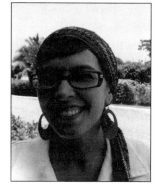

school when I spoke with her. Though she could have gone directly into medical school, she had taken a year of pre-med to improve her science skills. Cassandra's work with ELAM's student government led to a course on popular education being taught there and to some new electives being offered, such as Chinese medicine.

Cassandra felt a strong obligation to return to the United States to practice a Cuban-style medicine that emphasizes family medicine and gynecology. When she first came to Cuba after high school, she saw how people do not need many material possessions, but do need a sense of belonging and safety, which the island offers. Living with thousands of people from the Americas has been the most tremendous experience of her life.

KETIA BROWN

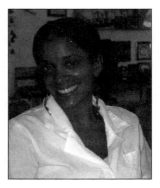

A thirty-year-old student from California, Ketia Brown had first heard of ELAM in 2003. She had wanted to go to medical school, but because of her interest in public health, not in the United States. ELAM was a perfect match. She had been teaching high school. Her mother was also a teacher and her father coordinated janitorial work. Ketia hoped, after getting her degree, to continue working with high school students and open a wellness clinic that would focus on the lifestyle changes needed for better health.

When I met Ketia, she was pouring energy into the Ghana Project. Medical brain drain is so drastic in Ghana that the country is left with one doctor for every 45,000 residents. The Ghana Project was one of the many projects designated as *Brigadas Estudiantiles por la Salud* (BES, Student Health Brigades), which ELAM students design and carry out themselves during summer vacation. The Ghana project emphasized traditional forms of medicine taught at ELAM and widely practiced in Africa. The 2010 phase of the Ghana Project began with ELAM students traveling to Ghana to meet with Cuban-trained doctors who were already there. The Project hoped to create an internship so that sixth-year ELAM students could complete their medical training in Ghana.

DENNIS PRATT

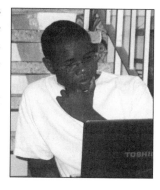

Dennis Pratt lived the first thirteen years of his life in Bo, Sierra Leone, where he spoke the regional Mende language as well as Krio. When civil war ripped the country apart and his cousins were killed, his family made its way to neighboring Guinea in 1997. In 2001, they moved to Jonesboro, Georgia, where his brother had been living. Studying medicine had been in Dennis's mind for years, but he could not bear the thought of graduating with a huge debt. In 2006, he looked up ELAM on the web. He applied in 2007 and began studying there the next year. Dennis took Spanish during his pre-med year. At twenty-six when I spoke with him, he was finishing his second year at ELAM.

Dennis planned to take board exams in the United States after graduating but would spend most of his time in Sierra Leone. Most communities are underserved in Sierra Leone, which has a national health care system that controls the hospitals even though there is also private practice. Sierra Leone has a good relationship with Cuba, and Dennis felt he would have no trouble practicing medicine there. He wanted to combine health education, pediatrics, and internal medicine.

LORINE AUMA

When I interviewed her, Lorine Auma was an eighteen-year-old pre-med student from Kisumu in western Kenya. She spoke Swahili, English, and Spanish and had long wanted to be a doctor. In high

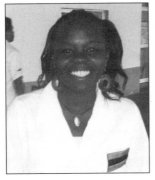

school, she had read an advertisement about ELAM and applied to the Kenyan Education Ministry. The Kenyan government selects students for study in ELAM but without the involvement of political parties.

Lorine's family had to pay for her transportation to Cuba, which meant she could visit them only once during her six years of study.

Her father, an accountant, and her mother, who sometimes worked as a printer, had been very happy that she would be going to Cuba. The Kenyan government gives students loans for medical school, which are reimbursed by paycheck deductions when they become doctors.

When she graduates, Lorine would like to specialize in orthopedics and psychiatry, but before then she was hoping to spend a summer in Ghana with the Organization of African Doctors. Lorine thought that ELAM offered a better medical education than she would have gotten in Kenya. Professors in Kenya have little direct contact with the students and rarely make multimedia presentations. At ELAM, she could listen to what professors are saying and ask them questions. Also, the professors often call on students in class. Lorine felt that the private university in Kenya was good, but it was far too expensive for her.

YELL ERIC

Yell Eric was from the city of Trindade in the island country of São Tomé and Príncipe, which is located off the coast of Central Africa. He spoke Portuguese and was learning Spanish during his pre-med year at ELAM. When Yell was eighteen, the government told him that, based on his grades and exam scores, he had been accepted for medical school, but they

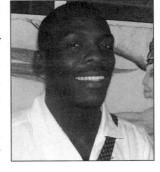

could not tell him where. Shortly before leaving home, Yell learned that he would be going to Cuba.

At ELAM, Yell found it a challenge to master the science courses in pre-med. Since there are plenty of general practitioners in São Tomé and Príncipe, he was planning to study a medical specialty; but he was not sure what it would be. Yell told me that he would be required to work for three years in a government job to pay back the cost of his transportation to and from Cuba.

KEITUMETSE JOYCE LETSIELA

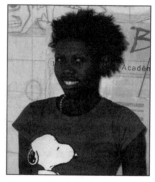

Keitumetse Joyce Letsiela, from rural Lesotho, was an eighteen-year-old first-year student when I interviewed her. She had applied to ELAM during her last year of high school, after talking with a doctor she knew and seeing an advertisement for the Cuban medical school. Her mother, a teacher, was both happy and worried that she would be studying so far away. The Lesotho government loaned her money for transportation, which Joyce would have to pay back after graduating.

Speaking only Sesotho and English, Joyce found ELAM difficult at the beginning, because she had to learn Spanish. She missed home but was becoming used to Cuba after getting to know other students from Lesotho and elsewhere. What she liked best about ELAM, which was her first choice for medical school, was meeting people from all over the world. She saw ELAM students as independent and serious. Since there was no medical school in Lesotho, the main option was studying in South Africa, but very few go because of the cost. Joyce said that there are only two doctors in the public hospital near her home. She would like to choose a specialty but had not yet decided what it would be.

Jonalisa Livi Tapumanaia

Twenty-two-year-old Jonalisa Livi Tapumanaia, from the island nation of Tuvalu,
may be among the first students to see
her homeland go underwater due to climate change. ELAM will make it possible
for each of the ten major islands in the
Pacific that comprise Tuvalu to have its
own doctor. At the time of the interview,
Tuvalu's few doctors were at the hospital
on the major island.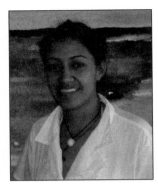

Jonalisa had graduated with a degree in marine science from the
University of the South Pacific in Fiji. Since she had had biology,
chemistry, and physics courses, her only concern in pre-med was
mastering Spanish. Jonalisa had heard about ELAM from the Ministry
of Health. The Tuvalu government recognizes medical degrees from
Cuba and was paying for her transportation, but it would cover only
one trip home during her six years of study. Her father, who ran a gas
station and food shop, and her mother, a court magistrate, did not
make enough to pay for additional trips.

Cuba is hotter than Tuvalu, and life is very different there. Jonalisa
had to get used to people kissing her on the cheek instead of shak-
ing hands. Tuvaluan women, unlike Cuban women, do not expose
themselves by wearing sleeveless shirts or miniskirts, and arranged
marriages are common. Jonalisa had been used to living in a thatched
roof home and going to school barefoot. Like most people in Tuvalu,
Jonalisa was a Methodist in the Ekalesia Kelisiano Tuvalu church. She
had heard that people in Tuvalu had once worshipped the trees, the
moon, and the stars, but that was not a part of her life.

Jonalisa told me that Western culture had profoundly changed life in
Tuvalu. This included providing three Cuban-trained doctors. But the
largest changes are due to climate change. Storms were getting worse. In
2008, a big wave hit one island and most people's belongings had been
swept away. The tide had gotten higher, land was being eroded, and one

of the smaller islands no longer existed. Rising sea levels had made one airstrip almost unusable. Those most worried about climate catastrophe were talking about migrating to Fiji or New Zealand.

Perspectives

Several themes run through these stories. All the ELAM students I spoke with shared a desire to provide medical care to people who otherwise might not receive it. There was no discussion about becoming wealthy, which is a highly unlikely outcome for an ELAM graduate.

Cuba's MGI medical model emphasizes family practice as the basis of holistic medicine. The excellent level of care that Cubans receive is largely due to the high number of family doctors in neighborhood *consultorios*. Nevertheless, a majority of students I spoke with were thinking about pursuing a specialty. This may appear to contradict the Cuban emphasis on general medicine, but it is understandable because of the severe shortage of specialists in so many of their countries of origin.

Many of the students I interviewed had aspired to be doctors early in their lives and later discovered ELAM. Others did not even consider the possibility of becoming a doctor until they heard of ELAM. The youngest student I spoke with was eighteen years old and the oldest thirty-one. The students from Africa tended to be the youngest, and those from the United States the oldest. The U.S. students had completed undergraduate studies, whereas students from Latin America and Africa had more often gone directly from high school to medical school.

The methods that countries use to select students for ELAM vary enormously. In some countries, political affiliations and recommendations are critical. In others, it is purely on the basis of grades. While most countries welcome students with Cuban medical degrees, some, such as Brazil, Honduras, and the United States, are more hostile. The medical association in Brazil would not recognize a degree from ELAM. The United States does nothing to help ELAM students and makes travel difficult. Honduran students trained in Cuba have been attacked back home. Most of the students I spoke with would have been unable to attend medical school without ELAM. This indicates that the shortage of doctors in impoverished areas has nothing to do with a lack of young people willing to become doctors and working in those communities. In fact, the shortage is due to the unwillingness of governments to provide adequate medical training.

WHERE WERE STUDENTS FROM?

My interviews with ELAM students were designed to capture a wide range of experiences and were not intended to be strictly representative of the school's students. However, the seven discussions with women and six with men approximates the gender breakdown of ELAM students in Havana, which in 2010 included 4,807 women and 4,868 men. They came from one hundred different countries, and about a third of them lived on the main ELAM campus near Havana.[2] In April 2010, ELAM students represented about half of Cuba's 21,018 medical students.

Though Africa was the continent with the largest number of countries (36) represented at ELAM, the 7,777 Latin American students from 15 countries comprised over 80 percent of students. Africa came next with 9.1 percent of students, followed by the Caribbean with 7.3 percent. Much smaller portions of students came from Asia (0.7 percent), Europe (0.1 percent), the Middle East (0.5 percent), Canada/United States (1.2 percent), and the Pacific Islands (0.7 percent).

Students at ELAM can directly observe how the MGI model of medicine has improved the health of Cubans—for example, by making Cuban life expectancy equal to that of the United States, despite the vicious U.S. embargo and Cuba's very low GDP (Gross Domestic Product). Rather than being an isolated progressive minority, ELAM students are surrounded by thousands of like-minded students from countries that suffer oppression in myriad ways. This is the social context where they spend six years studying the Cuban approach to health care. ELAM students are anything but passive observers; rather, they become active participants in creating a new global medical culture.

— 9 —

CUBA: THE NEW GLOBAL MEDICINE

uba is remaking medicine in a remarkable diversity of cultures—in Latin America, the Caribbean, Africa, Asia, and the Pacific Islands. Its efforts go far beyond providing medical care to other parts of the world as a Western approach might limit itself to doing. Instead, the Cuban project develops bilateral agreements with host countries to rethink, redesign, and re-create medicine.

John Kirk and Michael Erisman's book *Cuban Medical Internationalism* (2009) provides the most comprehensive documentation of the extent of this undertaking.[1] Since 1961, over 124,000 health professionals have worked in over 154 countries. In 2009, 24 percent of Cuba's 70,000 doctors were participants in health care "brigades" on international "missions." Though the majority of Cuban doctors travel to locations in the Americas or Africa, they have also provided relief: to Ukraine after the 1986 Chernobyl meltdown, Sri Lanka following the 2004 tsunami, and Pakistan after its 2005 earthquake. Cuba is establishing medical agreements with Laos, Kiribati, the Solomon Islands, Papua New Guinea, Vanuatu, and Tuvalu. By 2008, in addition to 11 million people in their own country, Cuban doctors were providing medical care for over 70 million people. "Almost 2 million people throughout the world, many of whom were probably children when they received help, owe their very lives to the availability of Cuban medical services."[2]

Venezuela has developed closer ties with Cuba than any other country and has received the most help from it. According to Steve Brouwer's deeply insightful *Revolutionary Doctors* (2011), over 14,000 Cuban doctors had come to Venezuela by 2009.[3] To date, Venezuela is the only country that has sought to reproduce the Cuban model on a national scale.

Examining projects in three other countries reveals some of the strengths and contradictions of Cuba's medical internationalism:

1. After participating in the emergency response to the 2007 earthquake in Peru, Cuban doctors faced multiple obstacles as they set up *consultorios* and a *policlínico* based on the Cuban model.
2. During relief efforts following the 2010 earthquake in Haiti, Haitian patients developed very different relationships with Cuban doctors than they did with those from the United States.
3. African and African-American medical students in Havana were working to blend Cuban medical approaches into traditional Ghanaian healing practices.

A POLICLÍNICO AND CONSULTORIO IN PISCO

On August 15, 2007, my daughter Rebecca Fitz and her partner, Ivan Angulo Torres, were vacationing in Arequipa, Peru. At 6:40 p.m. a magnitude 8 earthquake hit the town of Pisco in Ica province of Peru. Rebecca went back to Lima. However, Ivan, who had just completed his fourth year at the Latin American School of Medicine in Havana (ELAM), went to Pisco to help.[4] Soon, reports showed that over five hundred Peruvians had died, another 1,042 were injured, and over 100,000 would be left homeless.[5] The first international relief team to arrive was the Henry Reeve Brigade from Cuba. (Cuba's first response teams for international disasters are named after Reeve, a New Yorker who joined the Cuban fight for independence and was killed in battle in 1876.) The Brigade came with medicines, medical equipment (including autoclaves for sterilization), and tents for examinations and surgery.

Finding the Cuban doctors well organized and able to deal with the disaster, Ivan and other ELAM medical students devoted themselves to documenting the Brigade's work. The resulting twelve-minute movie, *Nuestra Misión* (Our Mission) shows remnants of the poorly constructed homes that crumbled in the quake and the makeshift thatched houses that replaced them. Many injuries were followed within a week by pneumonia deaths from crowding due to the cold weather. In their emergency tent hospital, Cuban doctors carried out 1,980 operations, ran 30,734 diagnostic tests, and performed 151,454 therapeutic treatments. Help arrived from the Peruvian government only when press cameras were rolling.[6]

As the response to the earthquake subsided, the Cuban doctors transformed the emergency tent hospital into the Pisco *policlínico*, which has medical exam rooms, a birthing room, a recovery room, and outpatient operating rooms. By far the rooms most in demand at the *policlínico* were for adult and child physical therapy. Three years later people were still suffering effects of the earthquake. When I visited the Pisco *policlínico* in 2010, its director, Leopoldo García Mejías, explained that then-president Alan García did not want any more Cuban doctors and that they had to keep quiet in order to stay in Peru. As is typical for Cuban medical directors, García had multiple international experiences, his first being in Honduras after Hurricane Mitch in 1998.[7]

Unlike in Cuba, there were charges for health care at the Pisco *policlínico*. It collected about 80,000 *soles* per year from patients, which it turned over to the Peruvian government for improvements.[8] But the improvements were not always forthcoming, which led to friction with the Alan García administration. By 2010, everyone knew that two hundred or so Cuban doctors were in Peru, making it possible for the *policlínico* to garner public support. Clearly, sustaining a health center was as much a political as a medical undertaking.

Peruvian doctors trained in Cuba set up three *consultorios* in Pisco, each with assistance from a nurse completing the last year of nursing school. Dr. Johnny Carrillo Prada and Dr. María Concepción Paredes Huacoto, Peruvians who received medical degrees at Cuba's ELAM, helped set up the Consultorio No. 2 in Pisco.[9] Carrillo and Paredes explained that the Peruvian health care system is not socialized medicine. For those who work, Peruvian social security takes money out of their paychecks for national health care, which has limitations, such as covering only two visits per month and only covering the "primary" illness for those with multiple health problems. A different system offers insurance to the poor and provides even less coverage. The *consultorio* must work within the framework of limited potential for reimbursement while attempting to see everyone who comes through the door. Consultorio No. 2 serves about 180 families; each pay one *sol* per month.

The backbone of the Cuban system of *medicina general integral* (MGI, comprehensive general medicine) is preventive community health care, with the *consultorio* as its building block. The doctor-nurse team lives in or near the *consultorio* where they work, so they are part of the community. Cuban *policlínicos* assist thirty to forty *consultorios* by providing services during off-hours and offering a wide variety of specialists. They coordinate community health programs and are a conduit between nationally designed health initiatives and their local implementation. By contrast, the Pisco *policlínico* provides a more limited array of services, not only because it has a smaller staff and is serving fewer *consultorios*, but also because it is not part of a system that requires patients to pay for health care.

There are other challenges to applying an MGI model in Peru. Cuban-trained doctors make home visits to everyone in the area of a *consultorio*. But in low-income areas of Peru, the only official-looking persons to come to the front door are usually the police. This means that medical staff have had to explain the central role of home visits. Since the country is rife with scam artists Peruvians were skeptical of a *consultorio* providing services at almost no cost, especially in an area as vital as medical care. In order to establish rapport with the neighborhood, the doctors had to work through businesses and schools where they could distribute health materials and provide physical exams. Perhaps the largest challenge has been Peru's weak educational system. The Cuban Revolution saw equality in employment, income, education, and medical care as proceeding together. The foundations of Cuban medical accomplishments are, on the one hand, a primary care system that prioritizes prevention and, on the other, scientific research scrutinizing the population's health needs. Thus, wiping out illiteracy has been vitally important to Cuban medical accomplishments. This makes it difficult to bring the model to a country where many cannot read and write.

One problem that Cuban-trained doctors have not had to face in Peru is a highly mobile population. In the United States, poverty often accompanies moving from home to home, which would make it very difficult to apply a model that assumes the doctor personally knows everyone in the community. In Pisco, however, even the poor tend to stay in the same home. *Consultorio* doctors are able to know their patients.

When Cuban doctors participate in a health brigade to another country, they respect its culture rather than impose their own social values. Without this approach, Cuban medical efforts in Peru never would have succeeded. Cuban doctors have to simultaneously practice medicine and adapt to a different society. The Alan García government, in power when the earthquake happened, merely tolerated Cuban medical efforts. A few days before being sworn in on July 28, 2011, as the new president of Peru, Ollanta Humala visited Cuban leaders in Havana and in his inauguration address, he pledged to eliminate "exclusion and poverty." As it turns out, Humala's government did result in better relations between Cuba and Peru in a number of areas.

DISASTER IN HAITI

When Joanna Souers was a nineteen-year-old in New York State, she decided to work with people who were down on their luck, a decision that would take her to Puerto Rico, Tanzania, Peru, Costa Rica, Mexico, Cuba, and Haiti.[10] After graduating with a major in pre-med in 2005, she went to Nicaragua to work on developing sustainable agriculture with Project Bona Fide. She lived on Ometepe Island, which mostly grew export crops like rice and coffee, leaving people without a sustainable diet.[11] Souers saw Nicaraguans who could not be treated by Western medicine because it is too expensive or inaccessible. People were more likely to use traditional medicine such as mango leaves for swollen joints and chamomile baths for fevers or coughs.

After Hurricane Katrina hit New Orleans in August 2005, Joanna went there and joined Common Ground Relief efforts in a nursing center to do support work. Cuba quickly mobilized 1,500 doctors on an airstrip ready to come to the aid of New Orleans. But Washington refused to accept its help. It left a lasting impression on Souers to know that the U.S. government prevented Cuba from helping thousands of New Orleans residents. She realized that Cuban doctors would have made an enormous difference in people's lives. Souers also observed that most of the hurricane relief aid went to the wealthier areas of the city where the storm caused much less damage.[12]

In 2006, Souers applied to go to medical school at ELAM. She began her studies in 2007 and had just finished the first semester of her third year when Haiti was devastated by an earthquake on January 12, 2010. The Haitian government estimated the death toll at over 300,000, with an additional three million people injured or left homeless.[13]

Souers took a semester off to work in the Croix-des-Bouquets field hospital about eleven miles from Port-au-Prince. The hospital had been established by the Henry Reeve Brigade. (The brigade was formed by the doctors who had been mobilized to aid New Orleans but were rebuffed by Washington.) She observed thirty to forty surgeries in the field hospital surgical tent, but mostly she assisted walk-in patients. Many of them had not been hurt by the earthquake but had other medical problems and had never seen a doctor.

Haitians traveled by foot to see Cuban doctors—some had to walk for hours from other towns. When they arrived, they found the Cubans living in tents not far from earthquake victims. The Cuban doctors felt the same heat, walked the same roads, heard the same nighttime noises, and smelled the same odors of injury and death as did Haitians. U.S. doctors, in contrast, typically slept in luxury hotels

in the Dominican Republic and were daily flown in and out by helicopter. Even if a disaster victim is grateful for assistance given, it was
clear that Cuban doctors were *of* the people and American doctors
were there *for* the people (and for U.S. TV cameras!). Though corporate television systematically ignored the work of Cuban medical
personnel, they treated vastly more patients than did U.S. doctors.
Hundreds of Cuban doctors practiced internal medicine, ob-gyn,
surgery, orthopedics, pediatrics, wound healing, and physical therapy day after day. By late March 2010, U.S. doctors had treated 871
patients, but the Cubans had treated 227,143.[14]

Being part of a Henry Reeve Brigade is stressful not only due to
the volume of patients, but also because a field hospital is so different from *consultorios* and *policlínicos* where most Cuban doctors work.
Souers was quick to point out that Cuban doctors in Haiti readily
adjusted to this stress, since most had already been on missions to
Sri Lanka, Mozambique, Venezuela, Honduras, or Angola.[15] Many
brigade members had previously served in Pakistan, where there
had been an earthquake disaster that resulted in similar pathologies.
Serving in international missions is some of the most prestigious
work that Cuban doctors can do.

The Croix-des-Bouquets field hospital had what was needed to
deal with most patients, though some of the more complicated cases
were sent to another hospital or to a location for treatment of chronic
diseases. Cuban doctors become resourceful at trying techniques that
may not appear in medical literature but work in disaster settings.
They may use tree limbs for splints or cinder blocks for traction.
Without having common anesthetics, Souers said, Cuban surgeons
had to rely on the local anesthetic bupivacaine and had to alter the
percentage solutions of dextrose to make it work for field surgery.
Doctors were always "on call" because patients with complex needs
frequently came in. Yet they would also do patient consultations.

A Cuban surgeon is trained to be a well-rounded specialist with the
full range of abilities needed in general medicine. A major strength of
Cuban doctors in a disaster setting is that they can make medical decisions quickly based on observation of patients. They typically rely on

much less expensive tests such as MRI, CAT scan, PCR (Polymerase Chain Reaction), X-rays, or ultrasound. Medical school teaches them to use basic lab tests and turn to X-rays or ultrasound only when it is necessary. Cuban doctors are familiar with the other tests and would use them if available but often make emergency decisions without them.

According to Souers, Cuban doctors possessing limited resources are not pressured to perform unnecessary tests. Also important is that Cuban doctors are not forced to constantly think about malpractice suits. Incompetent doctors are brought to trial, where their licenses could be revoked. Truly bad ones go to jail.[16] In contrast, U.S. physicians—trained to minimize exposure to legal risks—are often ill-prepared to deal with a massive disaster such as the Haitian earthquake.

Traditional and Western Medicine in Ghana

With the creation of Student Health Brigades (*Brigadas Estudantiles por la Salud,* BES), ELAM medical students could become protagonists in Cuba's international health care work, which I call the New Global Medicine. One of the most outstanding examples of BES work was the Ghana Project. Created by the Organization of African Doctors in 2009, it aimed to build closer ties between ELAM students and Cuban-trained doctors in Ghana.[17] ELAM students who carried out the Ghana Project formed the Yaa Asantewaa Brigade (YAB). Born in 1840, Yaa Asantewaa was a warrior queen famous for leading the Ashanti uprising against British domination in the early 1900s in what is currently Ghana.[18] In 2010, Omavi Bailey was one of six YAB members who went to Ghana, worked with traditional healers, and made contacts in order to further develop the project.[19]

As the report on their 2010 work describes, "In the initial phase of this medical mission the fundamental objective was to conduct an assessment of the health care resources and needs in the rural communities of Ghana's Volta Region."[20] This included strengthening working relationships with Ghana's Ministry of Health and local community leaders.

The students traveled to Logba, a small rural town in the Volta region, where they stayed in the guesthouse. As would be expected for students trained at ELAM, shortly after arriving they did an assessment of water systems and living conditions, including garbage disposal. For Cuban medical practitioners looking at basic public health issues, such as the quality of drinking water, is an indispensable part of evaluation. The YAB students also found that attending a large community funeral ceremony was important for understanding the village's culture and being accepted as family.

The Cuban MGI approach requires students at ELAM to study traditional and natural medicine, and roughly 85 percent of Ghanaians rely solely on traditional healers. Western medicine is unavailable, unfamiliar, and costly. Logba residents would have to travel at least thirty miles to see a medical doctor. Many Ghanaians do not receive conventional medical care because they cannot afford it. The YAB students reported that their own transformation toward understanding the culture of natural medicine was the most profound aspect of their trip to Ghana. Meeting tribal chiefs and being accepted by the village was critical, not just for obtaining information from villagers, but also for understanding how everyday life is part of the healing system. When I asked Omavi Bailey for examples of traditional healing methods, he mentioned massages being used for certain ailments and the employment of herbs to treat asthma. However, he emphasized that philosophical and spiritual dimensions of health and healing can transcend specific cures. These include cultural traditions such as not eating pork and counseling sick people concerning how to live better in order to avoid problems.[21]

The YAB students came to appreciate how the different spheres of life, rather than being divided from one another, are part of an interrelated whole. This holistic view led them to understand the importance of blending traditional and Western medicine in a way that makes health care not just affordable but also meaningful and culturally respectful of Ghanaians. Conceptualizing the wholeness of human health helped the Ghana Project transition from a focus on infectious disease to hypertension. When the students went to Ghana, they had a major interest in infectious diseases that plague Africa.[22] At the Logba clinic, they provided "primary medical attention to over 400 patients."[23] They observed traditional healers give consultations as they took vital signs and medical histories.

To their surprise, hypertension was rampant, with 59 percent of men examined having either high blood pressure, a history of mild stroke, or arthritis, while 46 percent of women had the same symptoms. Realizing that prevalent infectious diseases like malaria are well studied, they decided to shift the 2011–12 phase of the Ghana Project to investigating and treating hypertension.

Bailey observed that although Ghanaians were generally active doing manual labor, they still had hypertension. He wondered if their disconnection from traditional Ghanaian ways of living, adopting Western lifestyles, could be contributing to stress. There was also the possibility that the introduction of environmental toxins in Ghana might weaken the body's ability to cope with stress and indirectly lead to hypertension. Bailey hoped to look at all of these factors during future trips. But the most important question for him was whether traditional Ghanaian healers might already have treatments that were effective for hypertension.

At the time I spoke with Bailey, the students in the Ghana Project were planning to research hypertension and raise money to return. They were also going to improve their website so they could disseminate information more rapidly and do organization work requiring many phone calls. However, the U.S. blockade interferes with internet and phone connections in Cuba.[24]

For this reason, ELAM students have found that they need to do much of their organizing, especially making international connections, during summer trips to the United States. This is just one concrete example of how the U.S. blockade hampers Cuban medical initiatives and slows the improvement of global health.

Conceptualizing the New Global Medicine

In science, a theory or proposal is considered rigorous if it withstands multiple challenging tests. The MGI model of medicine withstood the test of Cuba's Special Period when, following the fall of the Soviet Union, oil imports almost dried up, the island's Gross Domestic Product plummeted, and 13 percent of the population became undernourished.[25] During this time, the United States sought to strangle Cuba by a series of laws that further hampered its ability to import goods, including pharmaceuticals.

Yet, despite these severe setbacks, the rate of infant mortality in Cuba continued to fall in the 1990s and it was able to provide medical assistance to several countries hit by hurricanes. Consequently, Cuba's MGI approach to health is perhaps the most rigorous metatheory of medicine on the planet today.

Focusing on the scale of Cuban international aid—whether measured in terms of number of emergency teams sent, doctors working overseas, medical treatments provided, or lives saved—might give the impression that any country could replicate its efforts if it dedicated enough resources to doing so. My research suggests otherwise—it is highly unlikely that the United States could provide the same degree of aid even if it wanted to. The quantity of assistance that Cuba has provided presupposes the social relationships of medicine embodied in the MGI model.

Understanding the international success of Cuban medicine requires perceiving it not as a quantity of things but as a dynamic, unfolding process of becoming. The New Global Medicine is not merely a set of people and instruments that one country bestows upon another, but rather a way of mobilizing and using those people and instruments. The New Global Medicine is anything but patients' sitting passively, waiting for governments to do good deeds. Instead, it depends on people participating in the creation and defense of health care institutions. The model is based on the realization that health care is simultaneously a human right and something that people define and build as they adapt techniques and knowledge to their own culture.

— 10 —

CHALLENGES OF THE TWENTY-FIRST CENTURY

Innumerable issues confronted the Cuban medical system as it moved into the second decade of the twenty-first century. This chapter looks at three of those distinct yet interlocking challenges. The first focuses on Venezuela and its relationship with Cuba during the *Barrio Adentro* programs. Cuba's own path went from being ameliorative to transformative. During the early years of the revolution, Cuban doctors brought care to those who had little to none before. By the middle of the 1960s medicine inside of Cuba began to change the relationship between healers and the healed. Even though its international missions often involved teaching medical skills to those where it went, it did not alter the medical systems of the countries it assisted. Venezuela became the testing ground for transforming medicine internationally.

Another challenge that interfered with inclusive health care was Cuba's own homophobia. A legacy of homophobia obstructed efforts to create a new culture. Any country striving to comprehend gender health must come to grips with experiences of those who have feared rejection their entire lives.

The third challenge was developing the ability to link medical research with popular mobilization to overcome dengue fever. This is a prototype of how poor countries can combat mosquito-borne illnesses. Even without massive wealth, a society that understands the fundamentals of disease can minimize dangers if its citizens are thoroughly involved in the campaign.

The chapter concludes with a summary of lessons learned by Cuban doctors from their first participation in Algeria through the turn of the century. Those lessons run the gamut from technical abilities through the creation of social and political relationships that enhance the utilization of those techniques.

REVOLUTIONARY DOCTORS IN VENEZUELA

As Venezuela became the first country that sought to reproduce the Cuban medical model on a massive scale, it has done so in ways that are unique in both form and process. Steve Brouwer's *Revolutionary Doctors* (2011), which documents that effort, is essential reading for anyone interested in how medical systems can be improved, even without access to the financial resources of the overdeveloped countries. Brouwer's insights show how medicine intertwines with national and international politics, and it builds upon the growing body of information about medicine in Cuba. Some of the best previous works on the subject include Linda Whiteford and Laurence Branch's *Primary Health Care in Cuba* (2008) and John Kirk and Michael Erisman's *Cuban Medical Internationalism* (2009). Together, the three books show how the Cuban model grew by responding to a series of contradictions.

The first problem was the enormous disparities in the quality of medical care available in the island in the 1950s. There were huge gaps between the care given to rich and poor, urban and rural, and light-skinned and dark-skinned Cubans. To correct this, the revolutionary government immediately began to increase the number of hospitals throughout the island. However, the expansion of access to medical care during the 1960s led to a second contradiction, leading Cubans to recognize that the best medical care would be preventive rather than hospital-based. As a result, the 1970s saw the introduction of polyclinics, each of which provided preventive care in the form of inoculations and education for twenty to forty thousand residents. (Today, each polyclinic serves approximately forty to sixty thousand people.)[1]

Cuba was probably the first country in the world to recognize that clinics, though invaluable, do not create the close contact between health professionals and patients that are essential for genuine preventive care. This was the third contradiction. The Family Doctor Program got going in the 1980s. That program was based on Basic Health Teams, which consist of a doctor and nurse pair living at a small medical office, or *consultorio*, in the community they serve. The most revolutionary aspect of Cuban medicine is that family doctors are responsible for everyone in a defined geographical area.

Unlike the first three contradictions, the crisis of the 1990s was of external origin. The fall of the Soviet Union, the crash of the Cuban economy, and the tightening of the U.S. embargo left the island with much less energy, food, and medicine. Hardships were extreme: young men lost 25 percent of their caloric intake and nutritional deficits led to 50,000 cases of optic neuropathy. Nevertheless, Cuba trained four times more doctors during this decade than it had during the 1970s. Amazingly, rates of infant mortality continued to fall.[2] *Policlínicos* and *consultorios* had become so much a part of Cuban life that the island was able to weather the economic crisis.

The fifth challenge was Cuba's understanding that socialized medicine could not be realized in one country alone. Though Cuba's international medical humanitarianism spanned fifty years of revolutionary change, it grew by leaps and bounds in the first decade of the twenty-first century. International medical brigades began responding to crises throughout the world and over 20,000 students from one hundred countries came to Cuba for medical education at no cost.

The Cuban concept of *medicina general integral* (MGI, comprehensive general medicine) defines the Family Doctor Program put into effect in the 1980s. That program builds close doctor-patient relationships by having doctors see patients in the morning at the *consultorio* and make home visits in the afternoon. The Venezuelan *Barrio Adentro* (Inside the Neighborhood) program is based on this concept of medical professionals living in the same communities as their patients. Fidel Castro and Hugo Chávez laid its foundations with an agreement signed in October 2000. The agreement had Venezuela pledging oil and other goods and Cuba's providing human resources: teachers, agronomists, and medical professionals.[3] Seventeen of 24 million Venezuelans had no regular access to medical care when Chávez took office in 1998. The first wave of two thousand Cuban doctors arrived to help extend care to every corner of the country in 2003. By 2009, fourteen thousand Cuban doctors had worked in Venezuela.[4]

Like the Cuban MGI model, the Venezuelan *Medicina Integral Communitaria* program (MIC, comprehensive community medicine) involves recruiting thousands of students who go to medical school for six years. They observe interactions between patients and doctors beginning in their first year of school. In addition to treating people in their communities, the MIC program trains doctors in village settings. Some Venezuelan students are already mothers, and Brouwer describes one who began medical school at seventy-one years of age.[5]

The first stage of the *Barrio Adentro* program, called Barrio Adentro I, began in 2003 with the creation of numerous neighborhood *consultorios populares*. In 2004, the Chávez government initiated Barrio Adentro II, which supported the mushrooming *consultorios populares* with a system of *Clinicas Diagnosticas Integrales* (CDIs, Comprehensive Diagnostic Clinics). The CDIs have a variety of specialists, analytic equipment, and treatment options not available in the neighborhood *consultorios*.[6] The following year saw the beginning of Barrio Adentro III, which attempted to overhaul Venezuela's complex maze of hospital systems. In 2007, Barrio Adentro IV established fifteen specialty hospitals.[7]

One of the most striking differences between the health care metamorphoses in Cuba and Venezuela is their disparate time frames. Each major shift in Cuban medicine marked a decade. By contrast, a year was devoted to the corresponding modifications in Venezuela, each forming a stage of the *Barrio Adentro* project. Brouwer describes the inevitable conflicts and problems accompanying such rapid transformation, which yielded impressive results in Venezuela despite the difficulties. It may be easy to understand that a course which took decades to chart out in Cuba could be re-created more rapidly in a new context. Perhaps more surprising is that the sequence of the stages could be reversed. That is what happened in Venezuela. It took three decades for Cuban medicine to evolve from focusing on hospital care and polyclinics before hitting upon the MGI concept of the Basic Health Team. Once the Cubans realized that a doctor-nurse pair living in the community should be the cornerstone of community health, the Venezuelans used it as the beginning point of the *Barrio Adentro* program. After massive expansion of *consultorios populares* as their first step, the Venezuelans built more clinics to strengthen neighborhood health and only then overhauled their hospital system (which was the Cubans' starting point). In effect, the Venezuelan process of reform proceeded in an opposite direction from what the Cubans had done.

Many other differences affected the ways the health systems in the two countries were transformed. With 11 million residents, Cuba has a much smaller population than Venezuela. The vast majority of opponents left Cuba after the revolution, and then it was able to develop a cohesive approach to health care. By contrast, Venezuela has a population that is more than twice as large, ample frontiers with neighboring countries, and has lived through the continued presence of large anti-revolutionary forces that use the mass media they control to denounce any progressive change.

Despite these differences, there are many parallels between revolutionary medicine in Cuba and Venezuela, beginning with the doctor-nurse teams in both countries living in the areas they serve. Like doctors in pre-revolutionary Cuba (and through much of Latin America) physicians trained in Venezuela before the Bolivarian Revolution were highly reluctant to practice medicine in poor barrios or rural areas. The revolutionary government needed to train thousands of doctors to go to the areas most in need. The beginning point of revolutionary medicine is a new generation of doctors motivated by revolutionary consciousness. These doctors work, not to become wealthy, but because they find their efforts rewarding and meaningful for their patients' lives.

Governments in both countries quickly increased spending on medicine in the poorest regions, resulting in rapid reductions in both infant mortality and infectious diseases as well as increased life expectancy. These improvements could only occur because Cuba and Venezuela realized that improving medical care presupposes simultaneous improvements in literacy, education, and housing. Like Cuba, Venezuela also put emphasis on preventive medicine. Not seeing patients until they are sick is symptomatic of "sickness-based" medicine, which is predominant in the United States. Brouwer's description of statistical charts on the walls of a *consultorios popular* in Venezuela made me remember the same types of charts I saw in a Havana *consultorio*. This way of charting behaviors that should change reflects the "wellness-based" medicine of doctors who are familiar with their patients because they interact with them informally throughout the year.[8]

As the United States moves toward the destruction of Medicare and other programs that are essential for healthy living (such as Social Security), international financial Scrooges demand "austerity measures" that would sacrifice the health of entire nations on an altar for the sake of bank security. Brouwer describes an alternative in Venezuela that is truly revolutionary because patients are anything but passive recipients of a benevolent government:

Each neighborhood of 1,500 to 2,000 people that wanted a Cuban doctor to serve them was expected to organize a committee of 10 to 20 volunteers from the community who would commit themselves to finding office spaces, providing sleeping quarters, collecting furniture and simple fixtures and feeding the medical providers.[9]

Venezuela is now emulating Cuba's example of training doctors from other countries at its medical schools.[10] If the Cuban MGI model has morphed into MIC in Venezuela, what new concepts could be born in other countries of Latin America, Africa, and the Caribbean? We can be sure that, if successful, they will not rely on the expensive technologies employed in Western "sickness-based" medicine. Equally clear is that they will not be static repeats of Cuba or Venezuela but rather dynamic reinventions of medicine for the different cultures they serve.

Marching Against Homophobia

At an open forum at the Medical University of Cienfuegos, Cuba, a young Honduran wearing the medical school *bata* (white shirt) stood up and told the audience:

> This discussion has changed my mind about homosexuality. Now I understand what my lesbian friend went through. When she graduated from medical school in Cuba, she cried. She told me that she could live her life the way she wanted to when she was in Cuba. But now she was going to return to Honduras as a doctor and would have to hide her lifestyle, hide who she is.

The forum was part of the 2012 International Day Against Homophobia and featured Mariela Castro, daughter of Cuba's then-president Raúl Castro, and director of the National Sex Education Center (CENESEX). Mariela Castro is internationally recognized for her successful fight to implement sex education in Cuban schools and her current struggle to have gay marriage legalized in Cuba. About five hundred people, including many medical students, attended the forum in Cienfuegos. I was part of a group of fifteen who came as part of the "Gender and Health Care" program offered by Medical Education Cooperation with Cuba (MEDICC).[11]

The day before, we had traveled by bus from Havana to Cienfuegos where preparatory activities were already underway. They included five "social network workshops." Our group broke up and picked work groups based on our interests: Gay Men, Men and Diversity,

Lesbians, Youth, or Transgender. The Men and Diversity workshop had been going on for a few minutes when I walked in. The group leader wrote on a large tablet, while group members shared stories of victimization as gay men in Cuba. The group was composed of about forty people, who related how they had been rejected, ignored, ridiculed, or attacked. We then divided into smaller groups to prepare role-playing skits that would depict hostility against gays expressed at home, work, education, or in the media. Group members willingly and eagerly expressed themselves. They were also learning how to run workshops in their own towns as a means of helping others articulate their feelings and share their experiences.

In some ways, these workshops were much like those in the United States. Even though the fast-paced and consonant-dropping Cuban Spanish was hard to follow, it was clear that an emotional intensity pervaded the room. Every lesbian, gay, bisexual, and transgender Cuban knows that from 1965 to 1968 homosexuals were grouped with counterrevolutionaries and sent to obligatory work duty with UMAP (Military Units to Assist Production). The scars remain, although the practice faded out by the 1980s and the massive HIV education campaigns in the 1990s treated homosexuality as a fact of life.

The next day the "March Against Homophobia" went down Cienfuegos's beautiful and historic Paseo del Prado. Just before it started, a British television crew interviewed our MEDICC coordinator, Anna Dorman. Several in our group recognized Mariela Castro and went to have their photos taken with her. While walking over to lead the parade, she motioned to Dale Mitchell (director of a Jamaica Plain agency that provides services to elders in their homes) and Barbara Chicherio (then president of the Green Party U.S.A.). They joined her in holding the multicolored gay banner at the head of the march, which seemed to stop at every other corner for press photos.

Two of the one thousand marchers towered on stilts above the rest. Soon, we were not just walking but chanting and dancing down Paseo del Prado, accompanied by drums and trumpets. A few marchers wore bright pink shirts. Others sported T-shirts with a double male insignia. One man, who must have been seventy or eighty, was overjoyed that people from the United States were a part of Cuba's gay rights parade. With perfect English and only a slight accent, he said that he had fought with the U.S. Army in the Korean War. There were at least as many onlookers as marchers. Many had a very doubtful, almost frowning look, but faces often turned to smiles as they waved to a marcher they knew. Not everyone smiled, though. Some were heard to make comments like "Why do they bring this crap here?" "Damn queers!" and "They will make our city look dirty."

The contradictions between past and present and between government policy and a recalcitrant social reality left a deep impression on all of us. Our MEDICC translator, Georgina "Yoyi" Gómez Tablo, said, "This is important to me—my best friend died of AIDS. This shows we are doing something right. It makes me proud of being Cuban. It is so good to be part of a large group in favor of human rights." The MEDICC medical consultant, Maricela Torres Esperón, added, "There is a tradition of machismo not just in Cuba but in all of Latin America. People should not be defined by their sexual orientation. I am glad that the government was in favor of the demonstration."

In combating homophobia, Cuba is undergoing a tremendous social transformation that could make it a model for all of Latin America.

After lunch, we heard Mariela Castro direct the open forum at the Medical University of Cienfuegos. Perhaps the most interesting aspect of the forum was that basic questions were so frequent. Many in the audience had internalized myths about homosexuality and wanted answers. They asked questions such as: "Why are some people homosexuals?" "Is homosexuality a disease?" and "Do we need to cure it?" Mariela Castro proved highly skilled at addressing their questions. One person asked how she could justify the cost of sex change operations given that Cuba has such extreme financial stress. She answered the man by illustrating how devastating it would be to spend your entire life feeling that you were in the wrong body: "How would you feel if you woke up one morning to find that you had large breasts? And how would you feel if your penis were to shrink up and become a clitoris?"

Another wanted to know why, as a heterosexual woman, she would be so passionate about sexual orientation. She responded that her mother, the late Vilma Espín, had founded and led the Federation of Cuban Women and devoted her life to promoting gender equality in Cuba. Extending that to full LGBT rights is Mariela Castro's way to honor her mother and honor the revolution.

We would not have been able to see any of this without the coordination of MEDICC, which does research and offers a wide array of programs to increase understanding of Cuban medicine. Our week-long program included five days of intense participation, learning, and conversation. We arrived in Havana and begin by interacting with staff at the semi-rural 4 Caminos University Polyclinic. After visiting a neighborhood doctor's office (*consultorio*) we heard a general overview of the way the Cuban medical system approaches gender and health issues.

These activities, typical of MEDICC's educational programs, were interactive and hands-on. A mix of lectures, tours, discussions, forums, marches and performances offers the wholeness of a gestalt that would be missed by experiencing one part in isolation. It concretizes the reality that medical care is not a static structure but is a dynamically unfolding and developing relationship between science, education, practice, and culture.

Understanding Cuba's approach to gender health makes one appreciate both the joys and difficulties that accompany changing gender roles in Cuban society. The International Day Against Homophobia is like the rebirth of a revolution that had failed in an important aspect of human respect. From the beginning, the Cuban Revolution worked to provide health care, housing, education, employment, and gender equality, considering these to be basic rights. At the same time the revolution's own actions reinforced the homophobia that it is now struggling against.

Cuba has learned from experience that gender health means placing emphasis on at-risk groups. For this reason, it has paid special attention to maternal and child health; those with high-risk pregnancies; and those with sexually transmitted diseases. Cuba has also learned that gender health requires an emphasis on preventive medicine through neighborhood *consultorios* and *policlínicos* as well as through traditional and natural medicine. Nevertheless, gender health must transcend (meaning including and going beyond) these existing institutions. Cuba has discovered that a revolution in health care is not complete if people are excluded from social acceptance due to their sexual orientation.

As many Cubans attempt to change its legal system to end discrimination against homosexuals, it is becoming a model for challenging *machismo* throughout Latin America. However, historically ingrained prejudices cannot be overcome by laws alone. In Cuba, the LGBT community is mobilizing and demanding an end to prejudice and exclusion. These efforts of the LGBT community to make itself visible are a necessary step toward closing the gaps in the medical system and fulfilling the humanitarian goals of the revolution. A revolution is nothing if it fails to be an ongoing process of social transformation.

COMBATING DENGUE FEVER

"I'm on *pesquizaje*," my daughter Rebecca told me, using the Cuban term for health canvassing. "All of the third-, fourth- and fifth-year medical students at Allende have our classes suspended. We are going door-to-door looking for symptoms of dengue fever and checking for standing water."[12]

As a fourth-year medical student at Cuba's Latin American School of Medicine (ELAM), she was assigned to Salvador Allende Hospital in Havana. It handles most of the city's dengue cases. Though Rebecca has done such canvassing before, this was the first time she has had classes cancelled to do it. It was very unusual for an outbreak of dengue, a mosquito-borne illness, to occur this late in the season. She remembered most outbreaks happening in the fall, being over before December, and certainly not going into January and February.

Groups of medical students were assigned to a block of about 135 homes, most having from two to seven residents. They tried to check on every home daily but did not see many working families until the weekend. The first dengue sign they looked for was fever. The medical students also checked for joint pain, muscle pain, abdominal pain, headache behind the eye sockets, purple splotches, and bleeding from the gums. What is unique about Cuban medical school is the way students are trained to make in-home evaluations that include scrutiny of potentially damaging lifestyles, such as leaving water containers uncovered so that mosquitoes can breed.

Dengue is more common in the Cuban cities of Havana, Santiago, and Guantánamo than in rural areas. Irregular supply of water to the cities means that residents store reserves in cisterns. But cisterns with broken or absent lids and puddles from leaky ones are prime breeding sites for the *Aedes aegypti* mosquito, the primary vector (carrier) of dengue.[13] There is a significant difference between dengue fever (DF, which can be painful) and dengue hemorrhagic fever (DHF, which is both painful and life-threatening). DF is a viral illness that usually lasts a week or more and is uncomfortable but not deadly.[14] DF has four varieties (serotypes). If someone who has had one type of dengue contracts a different serotype of the disease, the person is at greater risk for DHF. Early DHF symptoms are similar to DF: the person will become irritable, restless, and sweaty, but can also develop hemorrhagic shock and die.[15] DF can be so mild that many people never know they have it, but they can be at increased risk for the far more serious DHF. This is why the Cuban public health model of reaching out to people is important in preventing a deadly epidemic. There are no known vaccines or cures for DF or DHF. The treatment addresses the symptoms. With DHF, this includes dealing with dehydration and often giving blood transfusions in intensive care.[16]

Each year, there are over 100 million cases of DF, largely in sub-Saharan Africa, the Caribbean, Latin America, Southwest Asia, and parts of Indonesia and Australia.[17] Between 250,000 and 500,000 cases of DHF occur annually and 24,000 cases result in death. Dengue was not identified in Cuba until 1943. Epidemics hit the island in the period 1977–1978 (553,132 cases), in 1981 (334,203 cases of DF with 10,312 cases of DHF), 1997 (17,114 DF cases with 205 DHF cases), and in the period 2001–2002 (almost 12,000 DF cases).[18] As with all vector-borne diseases, the most important step is prevention via vector control. Unfortunately, climate change is making local conditions more suitable for the mosquitoes that are vectors for dengue. During the last half-century, Cuban health officials have calculated a thirty-fold increase of the *Aedes aegypti* mosquito, which is the main vector. Since the 1950s, the average temperature in Cuba has increased between 0.4 and 0.6°C. Cuban health officials are well aware that "increasing variability may have a greater impact on health than gradual changes in mean temperature."[19]

The Special Period of the 1990s was a very difficult time for Cuba. Soviet support, which included supplying oil, came to an abrupt halt; production of food and other articles plummeted; and illnesses increased. The 1990s were also a time when there was a rise "in extreme weather events, such as droughts, and . . . stronger hurricane seasons." Increases in climate variability meant warmer and rainier winters, that favor the spread of mosquitoes. Another consequence of climate change is "insults to the upper respiratory tract, increasing viral transmission, particularly among infants and children."[20] Medical students in Havana come from one hundred countries around the globe.[21] No matter what accent they have when speaking Spanish, they have no trouble getting into homes. In Havana, there is nothing unusual about a foreigner in a *bata* (white medical coat) walking through homes, poking into yards, and peering onto roofs to see if there is standing water. Always in need of extra cash, many Cubans carry out some kind of less than totally legal economic activity in their homes (such as having a nail parlor in the living room). But everyone, both residents and medical students, understands that the inspections are only for public health reasons, not to hunt down non-legal businesses.

Cuba has experienced more than half a century of campaigns that are precedents for the current mobilization against dengue. Soon after the 1959 revolution, Cuba organized the literacy campaign, which sent teachers and students to every corner of the island. Beginning in the 1960s, the Committees for Defense of the Revolution (CDRs) worked with thousands of trainers, who in turn trained 50,000 more

Cubans to teach the importance of polio vaccinations. Since 1974, Cuba has not had a death from polio. Likewise, every hurricane season, the neighborhood CDRs prepare to evacuate the elderly, sick, and mentally ill. The CDRs also actively encourage pregnant women to regularly visit their neighborhood doctor's office, and they patrol the community to enforce the ban on growing succulents that attract mosquitoes.[22] Campaigns of this kind have accustomed Cubans to having the government bring public health projects into their homes.

Cuba places a very high value on researching preventive medicine. MEDICC (Medical Education Cooperation with Cuba) *Review* is a peer-reviewed open-access journal that works to enhance cooperation among "global health communities aimed at better health outcomes." Cuban researchers have played a key role in developing the widely accepted model that explains how DHF is determined by "the interaction between the host, the virus and the vector in an epidemiological and ecosystem setting."[23] In Cuba, applying this model has led to the following conclusions: (a) the most important risk factor for getting DHF is having a second infection of DF, which is of a different strain; (b) being infected a second time with a specific sequence of DF strains places children at a higher risk for DHF than adults; (c) white Cubans are at higher risk for DHF than Afro-Cubans; but (d) those who already have sickle cell anemia, bronchial asthma, or diabetes are at even higher risk.

Cuban researchers openly discuss weaknesses in their health care system, and one Cuban study indicates that there could be a "marked undercounting" of dengue due to many cases falling below the radar. Since the study examined data from a period of "maximum alert," undercounting could be widespread. Cuba has discovered that the community must feel that the dengue control program belongs to them if it is to be successful and sustainable. Excellent research published in the Brazilian journal *Cadernos Saúde Pública* in 2009 looked at the importance of the "active involvement of the community" in dengue control. The authors felt that Cuba's outdoor spraying of adult mosquitoes "is of questionable efficacy." Instead, they focused on "the bad conditions or absence of covers on water storage containers" in the city of Guantánamo.[24] The study used sixteen neighborhoods as a control group that carried out the usual practices of home inspections, measuring the degree of mosquito infestation, and larviciding (applying chemicals to kill mosquitoes during the larval stage of growth). In contrast, the intervention group did everything that the control group did but added intense involvement by local activists. "Formal and informal leaders" of the community worked with health professionals "to mobilize the population and change behavior," such as covering water containers correctly, repairing broken water pipelines, and not removing larvicide. Measuring the number of mosquitoes in the two communities revealed dramatic differences between the control group and the one with activist involvement. The authors concluded: "Community-based environmental management integrated in a routine dengue prevention and control program can reduce level of *Aedes* infestation by 50–75%."[25] Rebecca told me that when medical students inspect the homes of Havana residents, they find that the overwhelming majority comply with public health policy. However, some do not: a few cannot afford the proper lid for cisterns; some have mental problems that limit their ability to cooperate; and a few just do not care. Cuban public health research helps to identify the barriers that communities need to overcome to protect themselves from disease.

Imagine that medical schools across the United States sent their students to survey living conditions of poor black, brown, red, yellow, and white people across the country to determine what causes elevated mortality rates. Imagine too that health care professionals throughout the world demanded that people in poor countries be spared the mosquito infestations, rising waters, droughts, floods, species extinctions, and all other manifestations of climate change and overproduction for the benefit of rich countries. Further, imagine that in place of the current sickness industry, we had a new medical care based on caregivers going to those who need help. Finally, imagine citizens welcoming health professionals to walk through their homes, because they have seen mobilization after mobilization improve their lives. In effect, this is to imagine a new society.

WHY IS CUBA'S HEALTH CARE SYSTEM THE BEST MODEL FOR POOR COUNTRIES?

The current debate over health care in the United States is largely irrelevant to charting a path for the poor countries of Africa, Latin America, Asia, and the Pacific Islands. That is because the United States squanders perhaps ten to twenty times what is needed for a good, affordable medical system. The waste is far more than the 30 percent overhead that goes to insurance companies. Other sources of inefficiency include over-treatment; making the poor sicker by refusing them care; creating illnesses; exposing people to contagion through over-hospitalization; and disease-focused instead of prevention-focused research.[26]

Poor countries simply cannot afford such an inefficient health system. Well over a hundred countries are looking to the example of Cuba, which has the same seventy-eight-year life expectancy as the United States and spends only 4 percent per person of U.S. health costs.[27] The most revolutionary idea of the Cuban system is doctors living in the neighborhoods they serve. This means that a doctor-nurse team is part of the community, and they know their patients well because they live at (or near) the *consultorio* (doctor's office) where they work. *Consultorios* are backed up by *policlínicos* that provide services during off-hours and offer a wide variety of specialists. *Policlínicos* also coordinate community health delivery and are charged with implementing nationwide health initiatives locally.

Cubans call their system *medicina general integral* (MGI, comprehensive general medicine). It focuses on preventing people from getting diseases rather than curing them after they are sick. This has made Cuba extremely effective in addressing everyday health issues. Having doctors' offices in every neighborhood has made prenatal care readily available, bringing the Cuban infant mortality rate below that of the United States and less than half that in the U.S. black population.[28] Cuba has a record unmatched in dealing with chronic and infectious diseases with amazingly limited resources. The country eliminated polio in 1962, malaria in 1967, neonatal tetanus in 1972, diphtheria in 1979, congenital rubella syndrome in 1989, post-mumps meningitis in 1989, measles in 1993, rubella in 1995, and tuberculosis meningitis in 1997.[29]

The integration of neighborhood doctors' offices with area clinics and the existence of a national hospital system mean that the country responds well to emergencies. Cuba can evacuate entire cities during hurricanes, largely because *consultorio* staff know everyone in the neighborhood and know who to call for help getting disabled residents out of harm's way. At the same time that New York City (which has roughly the same population as Cuba) had 43,000 cases of AIDS, Cuba had only two hundred AIDS patients.[30] Recent emergencies, such as outbreaks of dengue fever, have been quickly followed by national mobilizations. Perhaps the most amazing aspect of Cuban medicine is that, despite being a poor country, Cuba has sent over 124,000 health care professionals to provide care in 154 countries.[31] In addition to providing preventive medicine, Cuba sends response teams worldwide following disasters (such as earthquakes, hurricanes, and a nuclear meltdown) and has over twenty thousand students from other countries studying to be doctors at its Latin American School of Medicine in Havana.[32]

Synthesizing my own investigation and the work of others, I conclude this chapter by presenting ten general lessons that can be drawn from the Cuban health care experience. They form the basis of what I call the New Global Medicine and summarize what many authors have observed in dozens of articles and books.

First, it is not necessary that the initial approach to medical care be based on expensive technology. Cuban doctors employ whatever instruments are available, but they have an amazing ability to treat disaster victims through field surgery. They are also aware that most lives are saved through preventive medicine—including nutrition and hygiene—and that traditional cultures have their own healing practices. This contrasts sharply with Western medicine, especially as practiced in the United States, which uses costly diagnostic and treatment techniques as the first approach.

Second, doctors must be part of the communities where they work. For Cubans working abroad, this could mean living in the same neighborhood as a Peruvian *consultorio* or living in a Venezuelan community that is much more violent than a Cuban one. Alternatively, it could mean staying in a village guesthouse in Ghana or living in emergency tents adjacent to where victims are housed as Cuban medical brigades did after Haiti's 2010 earthquake. Cuban-trained doctors know their patients by experiencing their patients' communities. This differs sharply from U.S. doctors, who receive little, if any, training on how to assess their patients' living conditions.

Third, the MGI model focuses on relationships between people that go beyond a set of facts. To pass medical exams, students in the United States must memorize mountains of information that is of little importance to community health. By contrast, Cuban students learn what is necessary to relate to people in *consultorios, policlínicos*, field hospitals, and remote villages. Far from superfluous, Cuban courses that focus on people as bio-psycho-social beings are a critical part of the country's holistic medicine.

Fourth, the MGI model is not static but is evolving and unique for each community. Western medicine searches for the correct pill or surgery for a given disease. In its rigid approach, such research often has to discover a new pill for "side effects" of the first pill. By contrast, the MGI model relies on traditional medicine that has evolved in a given society over centuries and thereby avoids imposing a Western mindset and disease model.

Fifth, medical aid must adapt to the political climate of the host country. This means using whatever resources the host government can offer and accepting restrictions. A Cuban medical brigade may have a friendly reception, as occurred in Venezuela and Ghana, or face hostility, as happened in Brazil due to its Medical Association. Further, a friendly country can become hostile, as occurred in Honduras following the 2009 coup, or a formerly unreceptive country can become more welcoming, as happened in Peru with the 2011 election of Ollanta Humala to the presidency. This is quite different from U.S. medical aid which, like its food aid, is part of an overall effort to dominate the receiving country and push it into adopting a Western model of medicine.

Sixth, the MGI model creates the basis for dramatic health effects.
Preventive community health training, a desire to understand traditional healers, the ability to respond quickly to emergencies, and an
appreciation of political limitations give Cuban medical teams a track
record of astounding success. During the first 18 months of Cuba's work
in Honduras following Hurricane Mitch infant mortality dropped from
80.3 to 30.9 per 1,000 live births. When Cuban health professionals
intervened in Gambia, malaria decreased from 600,000 cases in 2002 to
200,000 two years later. And Cuban/Venezuelan collaboration resulted
in 1.5 million vision corrections by 2009. Kirk and Erisman conclude:
"Almost 2 million people throughout the world . . . owe their very lives
to the availability of Cuban medical services."[33]

**Seventh, the New Global Medicine can become reality only if
medical staff put healing above personal wealth.** In Cuba, being
a doctor, nurse, or support staff and going on a mission to another
country is one of the most fulfilling activities a person can do. Medical
fields attract an increasing number of students, despite the relatively
low salaries of Cuban health professionals. In the United States, there
are indeed some doctors who focus their practice on needy, low-
income communities that have the greatest need. However, there is
no political leadership making a concerted effort to get physicians to
put vocation above wealth.

**Eighth, dedication to the New Global Medicine is now being
transferred to the next generation.** When students at Cuban schools
learn to be doctors, dentists, or nurses, their instructors tell them
of their own participation in health brigades in Angola, Peru, Haiti,
Honduras, and dozens of other countries. Beginning with their entry
into medical school, students consider if they would like to practice
abroad and where they could go.

Ninth, the Cuban model is remaking medicine across the globe.
Though best known for its successes in Latin America, Africa, and the
Caribbean, Cuba has also provided medical assistance in Asia and the
Pacific islands. It supplied important aid to Ukrainians after the 1986
Chernobyl meltdown, to Sri Lanka following the 2004 tsunami, and
to Pakistan after its 2005 earthquake. Many of the countries hosting

Cuban medical brigades are eager for them to help rethink components of their own health care systems.

Tenth, the new global medicine is a microcosm of how a few thousand revolutionaries can change the world. One does not need vast riches, expensive technology, or a massive increase in personal possessions to improve the quality of people's lives. Revolutionaries who are dedicated to helping people and capable of learning from them can begin a rational employment of available resources that prefigures a new society. To a world threatened by imminent climate catastrophe, this kind of revolutionary activity is also proof that we can resolve many basic human needs without escalating carbon emissions.

Discussions of global health in the West typically decry the ongoing presence of controllable chronic and infectious diseases in poor countries. International health organizations wring their hands over the high infant mortality rates and lack of resources to cope with natural disasters in much of the world.[34] They are right to worry. However, such organizations typically ignore the one system that actually functions in a poor country, providing health care to all of its citizens as well as millions of others around the world. The conspiracy of silence surrounding the resounding success of Cuba's health system is egregious, and it casts doubt on the good intentions of such organizations.

How should progressives respond to this manufactured ignorance regarding the most plausible solution to global health problems? A rational response must begin with spreading the word about Cuba's New Global Medicine through every form of alternative media available. The message needs to be: Good health care is not more expensive—revolutionary medicine is far more cost effective than corporate-controlled medicine!

11

CUBA'S MEDICAL MISSION

When the Ebola virus began to spread through western Africa in fall 2014, much of the world panicked. Soon, over twenty thousand people were infected, more than eight thousand had died, and worries mounted that the death toll could reach into hundreds of thousands. The United States provided military support; other countries promised money. Cuba was the first nation to respond with what was most needed: it sent 103 nurses and 62 doctors as volunteers to Sierra Leone. With four thousand medical staff (including 2,400 doctors) already in Africa, Cuba was prepared for the crisis before it began: there were already nearly two dozen Cuban medical personnel in Sierra Leone. After an initial assessment, Cuba dispatched another 296 to Guinea and Liberia. Since many governments did not know how to respond to Ebola, Cuba trained volunteers from other nations at Havana's Pedro Kourí Institute of Tropical Medicine. In total, Cuba taught thirteen thousand Africans, sixty-six thousand Latin Americans, and 620 Caribbeans how to treat Ebola without themselves becoming infected. It was the first time that many had heard of Cuba's emergency response teams.

The Ebola experience is one of many covered in John Kirk's book *Health Care without Borders: Understanding Cuban Medical*

Internationalism. It has a very different focus than his *Cuban Medical Internationalism: Origins, Evolution and Goals,* coauthored with Michael Erisman in 2009.[1] That book was a definitive work on the political history of Cuba's medical involvement across the globe. *Health Care without Borders* provides updates on the recent expansion of Cuba's programs, with a focus on the politics of international medical cooperation.

Cuba's most persistent difficulty in developing international medical policy has been the intense hostility it faces from some other countries' governments and medical associations, including those in the United States. As a psychologist, I use the term "neglect projection" to encompass several of these attacks on Cuban humanitarianism. The term "projection" describes individuals who attribute their own unacceptable thoughts or impulses to another. Political projection would be a country attributing its own reprehensible action to another government. Medical neglect projection against Cuba takes a variety of forms. Medical associations in several Latin American countries have displayed intense hostility toward Cuban doctors, accusing them of taking jobs from the country's own doctors; coming to another country just to spread propaganda; being underqualified; and not providing sufficient follow-up care.

The claim that jobs are being taken away from doctors in Brazil or Venezuela is belied by the fact that Cuban medical staff go to poor and rural areas where native doctors in those countries will not work. The Chávez government began the first *Barrio Adentro* (Inside the Neighborhood) program in 2003, to provide community medicine to poor and working-class Venezuelan districts. A call went out for Venezuelan doctors to participate; only fifty volunteered. It was this pathetic response that led Cuba to deploy over nine thousand of its own medical personnel by the end of that year. After *Barrio Adentro* began, the Venezuelan Federation of Medicine (FMV) demanded that Cuban doctors be expelled, partially because they were accused of spreading leftist propaganda. Yet unlike the ultra-politicized FMV, Cuban doctors have been trained to not meddle in the politics of any country where they are serving. This is critical for medical agreements with countries that, unlike Venezuela, have a right-wing government as well as right-wing doctors.

Medical associations in Costa Rica and Chile have charged that students trained to be doctors in Cuba scored lower on qualifying exams. This overlooks the unique focus in Cuban medical education on community health in distressed and rural areas, family medicine, and disaster management. Kirk reports that one question Cuban doctors often pose to their students is: "What would you do and how would you make the diagnosis if you were working in the middle of the Amazon and did not have access to any diagnostic tests?" Cuban doctors aim to diagnose over 80 percent of medical problems through examinations and detailed histories. The Cuban system has done exceptionally well at lowering infant mortality rates and improving other health indicators, meeting or exceeding results of more richly resourced systems. Instead of asking how students trained in Cuba perform on tests in other countries, it would be more useful to ask how graduates from Costa Rican or Chilean medical schools would perform on examinations in Cuba which emphasize practical over esoteric skills.

Perhaps the wildest accusation hurled at Cuban doctors has been that ophthalmologists in *Barrio Adentro* leave patients at risk if they are not present for postoperative complications. In fact, Cuban doctors have more staying power in distressed communities than do those making the charge. When Cuban doctors rotate home, other ophthalmologists from the island replace them.

The other major form of neglect projection has been to ignore or minimize the significance of Cuba's emergency response teams for floods, earthquakes, hurricanes, tsunamis, volcanoes, epidemics, and the Chernobyl meltdown. These stories rarely appear in the corporate media, despite dozens of Cuban life-saving interventions. Many Americans first learned of Cuba's disaster relief teams from news photographs of the 1,586 doctors waiting to leave Havana for New Orleans after Hurricane Katrina in 2005. Not only did President Bush refuse the offer; when U.S. State Department spokesman Sean McCormack thanked fifty organizations and countries for offering assistance, Cuba was noticeable by its omission.

Five years later, Haiti was not at all reluctant to accept Cuba's help following the country's devastating earthquake. Cuba was the key provider of help, since it had had so many medical personnel in Haiti since 1998. Over the years, 6,000 Cuban medical staff have treated over three million Haitians. Cuba also had previous emergency experience in Haiti, having sent a medical brigade during the massive flooding of 2004. Within a month of the 2010 earthquake, many foreign emergency teams had returned. But 600 Cubans and 380 Haitians trained in Cuban medical schools remained. In October 2010, Haiti was hit by the first cholera outbreak it had seen in over a century. Had Cuba not been in the habit of staying in a country after the initial excitement of disaster relief, and if it had not been teaching Haitians preventive medicine, the cholera death toll would have been much worse.

Though Cubans were in Haiti before the earthquake, provided the quickest and most professional emergency assistance, and remained long after the earthquake was history, Spain's leading paper, *El País*, omitted Cuba from its list of countries that provided help. In the United States, a 2012 study by Harvard Medical School failed to mention Cuba's contribution. Fox News actually criticized Cuba with the astounding claim that it failed to provide assistance. Meanwhile, the twenty-two thousand U.S. personnel in Haiti were almost entirely deployed by the military. Not only did U.S. doctors reach Haiti later and depart sooner than those from Cuba; they did not stay where Haitian victims huddled. After working hours, they tended to return to luxury hotels, while Cuban doctors lived in the communities of the Haitians they treated.

Kirk uses the term "disaster tourism" to describe the way that many rich countries respond to medical crises in poor countries. Many go to disaster areas, he writes, "to have an 'experience' rather than provide meaningful assistance to those affected."[2] Many end up getting in the way of serious rescue work. The approach of Cuban doctors stands in stark contrast to disaster tourism. Cubans have extensive training in intercultural disaster response. They build on the experience of thousands of medical staff who have already worked in poor countries. Cuban response teams or replacement staff stay in afflicted countries for months or years, helping to develop programs of community medicine and preventive health.

In many ways, Venezuela is a prototype of Cuban intervention. It began with Cuban assistance during the flooding of 1999, the year following Hugo Chávez's election as president. The first medical cooperation agreement was signed in 2000, amid widespread opposition by the Venezuelan right. The hostility greatly diminished as Venezuela's rate of infant mortality per thousand live births dropped from twenty-five in 1990 to thirteen in 2010. Huge numbers of Venezuelans have received treatment from Cuban or Cuban-trained doctors. Indeed, the greatest change in recent years has been Venezuela's taking over much of the care and training formerly provided by and in Cuba.

Misión Milagro (Miracle Mission), well-known for restoring sight to over three million people, began in Venezuela by accident. In 2004, Venezuela and Cuba were partnering in a program to teach literacy to eight million people when they realized that a major reason that many could not read was poor vision. Patients from Venezuela and throughout Latin America began flooding into Havana for eye surgery. The second stage of the program saw Cuba training Venezuelan and Bolivian doctors to perform eye surgery for their own and neighboring countries. *Misión Milagro* has been widely acclaimed for achieving such a great impact on so many lives at such a small cost. Much of the blindness in Latin America is preventable, often caused by living conditions such as contaminated water, malnutrition, and inadequate access to health care. Being blind is vastly worse in a poor country than in a rich one: families have few resources to spend on blind relatives, who become a burden on the family and face a life expectancy half that of the general population.

Health Care without Borders ties the issue of blindness into the first great investigation of its kind regarding disabilities. The family burden factor is why the handicapped or *discapacitados* are often referred to as *minusválidos* (those of lesser value). Meeting the needs of disabled people might seem routine in the United States, but it is highly unusual in impoverished countries. Many millions of poor

Latin Americans were amazed to find Cubans working with their government to address their needs. Some had to be reached by helicopter, donkey, or canoe. In Bolivia, 101 surveyed communities were so remote that they did not appear on any map. By 2013, hundreds of thousands of those surveyed in Cuba, Venezuela, Ecuador, Nicaragua, Bolivia, and Saint Vincent and the Grenadines had received concrete support such as wheelchairs, walkers, hearing aids, and prosthetic limbs.

Though most of what Kirk addresses are new twists on recognizable themes of Cuba's medical internationalism, he also brings to light areas likely unfamiliar to many readers, including Chernobyl and the south Pacific. The April 26, 1986, meltdown at Chernobyl occurred only a few years prior to the collapse of the Soviet Union, forcing Cuba to pay a high price for its humanitarianism. Cuba opened its doors, hospital beds, and a summer camp to twenty-five thousand Ukrainians, mostly children. Many had severe injuries or chronic pathologies. Some stayed in Cuban hospitals for months or years. In October 2011, Ukrainian President Viktor Yanukovych expressed his gratitude and promised to pay the full cost of treatment. Ukraine never got around to paying Cuba. The cost of medicine alone was estimated at $350 million.

The island nations of the south Pacific offer Cuba no strategic advantage, virtually no trade, and no investment opportunities. Yet Cuba has sent hundreds of medical professionals to the region, which in turn has sent hundreds of its students to train as doctors in Havana. Cuba helped set up a small medical school in Timor-Leste, which is now training doctors for other Pacific island nations. The fact that half of Cuban doctors are women has been very important in Java, where Muslim women are highly reluctant to be examined by a man.

Kirk's story of Cuba's research on medical biotechnology is the chapter that most intrigues me (though it may distress many others). As a resident of St. Louis, a veritable plantation of Monsanto (now Bayer), I have participated in and organized dozens of demonstrations at the company's world headquarters, as well as forums and conferences. It is necessary to compare the use of biotechnology by global corporations with that of Cuba to decide if they are basically the same or fundamentally different.

Technologies have various effects when introduced. Some, such as antibiotics, are positive, even if their ultimate goal is corporate profit. Others undermine organized labor: a classic example is the new molding machine adopted by the Chicago McCormick manufacturing plant in the mid-1880s. It could be run by unskilled workers, who promptly replaced the skilled workers of the National Union of Iron Molders. Still other technologies destroy small competitors so that large companies can better control the market. No case is clearer than the use of genetically modified organisms (GMOs) in agriculture. By use of market control (that is, making non-GMO seeds unavailable), financial terrorism (such as lawsuits against resistant farmers), and the pesticide addiction treadmill, GMO giants such as Monsanto have increased the cost of food production. This destroys the livelihood of small farmers across the globe while transforming the large farmers who remain into semi-vassals of these multinational lords of seeds and pesticides.

In using new technologies to attack labor or gain market control, capital is willing to create inferior products. McCormick used molding machines that produced inferior castings that cost consumers more because they were an invaluable weapon against the union. Likewise, GMOs in agriculture result in lower-quality food. Since two-thirds of GMOs are designed to create plants that can tolerate poisonous pesticides such as Roundup, pesticide residues increase with GMO usage. GMOs are also used to increase the production of corn syrup which sweetens a growing quantity of processed foods, and thereby contributes to the obesity crisis. At the same time, uniform food engineered to survive transportation and have a longer shelf life contains less nutritional value. The use of GMOs in corporate agriculture is one of the largest contributing factors to the phenomenon of people being simultaneously overweight and undernourished.

How do these disastrous effects of new technologies in corporate agriculture compare with Cuba's use of biotechnologies in medicine? Kirk convincingly argues that Cuba has produced new medicines that improve people's lives while sharing its biotechnology knowledge with other countries, in ways that empower rather than subdue them. Even a partial list of drugs developed in Cuban laboratories is impressive. The use of Heberprot B to treat diabetes has reduced amputations by 80 percent. Cuba is the only country to create an effective vaccine against type-B bacterial meningitis, and it developed the first synthetic vaccine for Haemophilus influenza type B (Hib), which causes almost half of pediatric meningitis infections. Cuba has also produced the vaccine Racotumomab against advanced lung cancer and has begun clinical tests for Itolizumab to fight severe psoriasis.

Patents for these and the vast number of other medical innovations are held by the Cuban government. There is no impetus to increase profits by charging outrageously high prices for new drugs, so these medications become available to Cubans at much lower cost than they would in a market-based health care system like that of the United States. This has a profound impact on Cuban medical internationalism. The country can provide drugs, including vaccines, at a cost low enough to make humanitarian campaign goals abroad more achievable. Using synthetic vaccines for meningitis and pneumonia has resulted in the immunization of millions of Latin American children.

Cuba's second phase of medical biotechnology is also unknown in the corporate world. This is the transfer of new technology to poor countries, so that they can produce drugs themselves. Collaboration with Brazil has resulted in meningitis vaccines at a cost of 95¢ rather than $15 to $20 per dose. Cuba and Brazil are working together on several other biotechnology projects, including Interferon alpha 2b for hepatitis C, and recombinant human erythropoletin (rHuEPO) for anemia caused by chronic kidney problems.

Kirk's discussion of agricultural biotechnology is limited to anti-pest poisons such as BioRat, sent by Cuba to Peru to fight an outbreak of bubonic plague by killing rats. BioRat is supposedly safe because it breaks down. However, Monsanto also claims that Roundup poses no threat because it "breaks down," but the resulting chemicals are highly toxic. The history of pesticides and psychotropic drugs that are claimed to be "safe," or to have only minimal side effects, and are then found to have severe consequences, is a long and tortuous one. Let us just say that the jury is still out on Cuba's use of toxins (including those developed with biotechnology) to control pests.

No country, even one whose medical policies have saved millions of lives, should get a pass on a potentially negative practice. Every new social and technological change should be open to scrutiny and com- radely criticism. Cuba has certainly made errors that could damage public health. Its gravest mistake, one that was more serious than all others combined, was the decision during the 1980s to build a nuclear power plant. That project was thwarted by the collapse of the Soviet Union and a consequent loss of funding; but if the plant had been built, it would not have been healthy, to say the least, for children and other living things on the island to risk a Chernobyl or a Fukushima. Another regrettable policy is Cuba's almost 1950s approach to mari- juana. Since it is one of the cheapest weeds to grow and could have a large variety of medical uses, Cuba is currently missing out on an opportunity to contribute to many low-cost treatments.

While we should not ignore these problematic decisions made by Cuba, they are vastly outweighed by the nation's contributions to global health. *Health Care without Borders* thoroughly documents how they extend beyond specific interventions to encompass the transfer of technology and the design of new health systems. How different this is from what is happening to drug costs in the corpo- rate world! For example, Rodelis Corporation obtained the rights to Cycloserine, one of the few antibiotics available to combat drug-resis- tant tuberculosis, and raised its price by 2,000 percent, so that a full treatment now costs $500,000.

In October 2015, it came to light that the Trans-Pacific Partnership (TPP) would extend the length of patent protection for pharmaceuti- cals to twelve years. During that time, cheaper generic alternatives to brand-name drugs could not be sold, leaving thousands, perhaps mil- lions, of people in the twelve TPP countries unable to afford critical medications. Such trade deals reveal drug companies as having the warmth and compassion of a school of leering sharks about to begin a feeding frenzy. The path that Cuba is forging leads in the opposite direction from that demanded by production for profit.

12

MEDICINE IN CUBA AND THE UNITED STATES

An excellent account of current community medicine is Conner Gorry's "Cuba's Family Doctor-and Nurse Teams: A Day in the Life."[1] It coincides quite well with my observations of a *consultorio* published six years earlier by *Monthly Review*.[2] Gorry combines data regarding health care with personal observations of social interactions (which are often omitted from analyses of medical systems). Each *consultorio's* doctor/nurse team is responsible for up to 1500 patients. The 12,833 family doctors in Cuba (one per 127 inhabitants) typically know each patient by name. Though some doctor-nurse teams live on the second and third floors above their office, more often they live within a block or two of it.[3]

Each of Cuba's 451 *policlínicos comunitarios* directs the work of up to 30 *consultorios*, providing services for 20,000 to 60,000 patients. The "polyclinics offer diagnostic procedures, laboratory testing, dentistry, physical therapy, natural and traditional medicine consultations and primary care specialties such as internal medicine, pediatrics, psychiatry and ob-gyn."[4] The Havana polyclinic I visited similarly had rooms for various services: admission, observation (to determine if hospitalization was necessary), autoclave, laboratory, vaccination, X-ray, optometry, ophthalmology, ob-gyn, family planning, ultrasound, menstrual regulation, mouth diseases, podiatry, psychology, social work, bone specialties, speech therapy, physical therapy, adult gym, children's gym, acupuncture, massage therapy, reflex therapy, electromagnetic therapy, mud therapy, and heat therapy.[5]

Students at ELAM explained to me that *consultorios,* which are designed to address 80 percent of medical issues, will refer patients with more complex problems to polyclinics. Polyclinics also deal with problems that arise when *consultorios* are closed. Higher levels of care continue to be addressed by hospitals, specialty hospitals, and facilities such as *casas para ancianos* (nursing homes) and maternity homes for women with high risk pregnancies. MINSAP (Cuba's Ministry of Public Health) oversees relationships between these facilities, health-related schools, and research institutes. MINSAP also establishes programs, national priorities, and health care guidelines.[6]

Each *consultorio* occupies a pivotal point for the larger system since its staff completes the Continuous Assessment and Risk Evaluation (CARE) form which determines the level of follow-up for each patient. These forms are used to decide which group each patient belongs to:

I. Healthy individuals;

II. At-risk persons who could develop health problems from risk exposure;

III. Sick persons, including those with chronic diseases; or,

IV. Disabled or incapacitated persons.

Family doctors and nurses are required to reassess those in Group I annually, Group II and IV twice per year, and Group III three times per year. These are minimal standards for visits which health professionals can choose to conduct more frequently. *Consultorio* Dr. Martha Díaz told Gorry that "I can't go six months without visiting my Group IV patients—disabled and homebound people. We visit them at least three times a year. And if one of our patients in Groups I, II or III experiences a change in their health, we'll see them more often than required—either here in our office or in their homes."[7]

Knowing that doctors must visit patients in both locations, I asked Dr. Alejandro Fadragas Fernández how he got to patients' homes. He looked at me like I was unbelievably ignorant for asking such an obvious question while replying, "I walk there." I explained that I wanted to ask my students in the U.S. how many times a family physician had walked to their home in order to contrast Cuban and American medicine.[8]

Gorry describes how *consultorio* walls have health posters and frequency tabulations of patient problems.[9] Similarly, I observed the *consultorio* tabulation of problems including "*Hab. De Fumar* (smoking habit), *Sobrepeso* (overweight), *Hipercolesterolemia* (high cholesterol), *Alcoholismo, Sedentarismo* (being sedentary, as in "couch potato), *Suicida,* and *Droga* (drug usage). I was impressed that the office included being sedentary as a health risk right between alcoholism and suicide. The *consultorio* walls also included the names of the three doctors and two nurses assigned to it (some professional staff work primarily at a *policlínico* with some time at the *consultorio*), and assigned medical students that ranged from first year ELAM students to an intern.[10]

The structure of a medical system is not separate and distinct from the social relationships fostered by that structure. A facet of the Cuban system that outsiders, especially Americans fishing for something to criticize, are likely to miss is that doctors' and nurses' living in the community they serve engenders a much closer relationship between professionals and patients. As Dr. Díaz told Conner Gorry, "We have a medical culture that promotes a warm, affectionate doctor-patient relationship: greeting patients by name and with a kiss on the cheek, holding their hand and having them sit beside rather than across the desk from us."[11]

Consultorio staff devote special attention to all at-risk persons, including pregnant women, infants and children, the elderly and those with any physical or mental disability. Physicians note whether each new mother is breastfeeding. A widely distributed booklet lists the first challenge to be met in child health care is "Promoting exclusive breastfeeding in children under six months and complementary breastfeeding in up to two-year-old children."[12] Home visits alert professionals to changing health care needs as children become adolescents, as mature adults become elderly, and if workers become injured on the job. Each *consultorio* is closely linked to a polyclinic (by way of doctors' working shifts at both), hospitals (since doctors visit patients and are part of planning for returning home), and teaching institutions (as they supervise students during their rotations).

The family doctor and nurse at each *consultorio* are part of the polyclinics' Basic Work Group (BWG) which also includes "an internist, pediatrician, ob-gyn, psychologist, nutritionist, and social worker.[13] The BWG both works with patients individually and collectively evaluates services and alerts staff to potential problems. The effectiveness of the Cuban health system is largely due to the interconnectedness of its components, totally unlike U.S. health care where services are not only disconnected but regularly go out of business and are replaced by other profit-seeking entities.

The Cost of U.S. Health Care

There is a growing body of literature demonstrating the increasing cost of U.S. medicine is in comparison with that of other countries. Some of the articles aim to show that National Improved Medicare for All (NIMA) would not increase the cost of care. Among them, a 2018 article in *The Nation* by Woolhandler, Himmelstein, and Gaffney points out that reductions in insurance premiums and out-of-pocket payments would more than offset any rise in taxes, resulting in an average savings of $6,000 per person and a total savings of $2 trillion over a decade.[14] Another study estimated that NIMA would reduce federal health care spending by $5 trillion over a decade and save 10 percent of total costs each year.[15] Comparative research of this kind almost exclusively explores how medical spending in the United States "can be brought in line with other wealthy countries."[16] For example, a Commonwealth Fund report contrasts the United States' spending with that of ten other rich countries (France, Australia, Germany, Canada, Sweden, New Zealand, Norway, the Netherlands,

Switzerland and the UK). It found the United States to have the most costly system in the world, despite very poor outcome measures.[17] A typical finding is that by David Rosen who noted that in 2013 the U.S. was spending $8713 per person annually on medical care while other Organization for Economic Cooperation and Development (OECD) countries averaged less than half as much—$3,453.[18] Pete Dolack looked at 2011 to 2016 figures from the period 2011–2016 and found that the average per capita health care spending in Britain, Canada, France, and Germany ($4,392) to be less than half that for the U.S. ($8,924)—he estimated that the annual cost for the Unites States not having a NIMA system was $1.44 trillion.[18]

Comparisons of U.S. health care costs to those in less wealthy societies, however, are much less common. Why not consider the possibility that other rich countries could also be wasting enormous resources on health care? In fact, a better comparison for potential savings would be Cuba, which despite being a poor country has indices of life expectancy and infant mortality similar to those of the United States. An Associated Press report found that, at the same time that the daily cost for inpatient hospital stays in the United States was $1,944, it was $5.49 in Cuba. The cost of hernia surgery in Cuba was $14.59 compared to the U.S. figure of $12,489; hip-fracture repair costs in Cuba were $72.15 compared to the U.S. figure of $14,263; and kidney transplant costs in Cuba were $4,902 compared to the U.S. figure of $48,758.[19] The article also points out that Cubans bring their own bed sheets, food, and water to the hospital. From my own visits to hospitals, I have seen how Cuban families are expected to launder the sheets and clothes of hospitalized relatives. In contrast to U.S. hospital rooms that might come with a color television receiving more than five hundred channels, Cuban hospital rooms, which are devoid of television, could appear bare. A 2005 study based on data from the World Health Organization noted that Cuba was spending $193 per person annually while the United States' annual per person costs were $4,540.[20] Similarly, in 2009, Kirk and Erisman found "the United States spending almost 20 times more per capita on health care than Cuba does . . ."[21] In 2018, Cuba was spending $431 and the

United States $8,362 per person annually on medical care.[22] For over a decade Cuba has been spending about 4 to 5 percent per person on health care of what the United States spends. The most important reason for this enormous disparity is that the sickness industry in the United States produces immense waste.

INSURANCE FRAGMENTATION

The most often cited reason for this waste is the parasitic nature of the insurance industry which both takes its own cut from the health care pie and geometrically increases the amount of paperwork for every other portion of the system. As the *Dollars and Sense* website points out:

> the U.S. has the most bureaucratic health care system in the world, including over 1500 different companies, each offering multiple plans, each with its own marketing program and enrollment procedures, its own paperwork and policies, its CEO salaries, sales commissions, and other non-clinical costs—and, of course, if it is a for-profit company, its profits.[23]

Each year the army needed to administer the labyrinth of health care plans increases in size. Steffie Woolhandler has calculated that administration eats up fully 31 percent of health care costs. In part this is because insurance companies competing in the market have duplicative claims-processing facilities and must keep track of a variety of approval and co-payment requirements.[24] According to economist Dean Baker, not only must care providers hire staff to cope with the huge number of different forms and billing practices but "employers who provide health care benefits need to devote staff time and/or hire consultants both to select and administer plans and to assist workers in making claims and choosing plans."[25] Health economist Austin Frakt has cited evidence that "billing costs primary-care doctors $100,000 apiece and consumes 25 percent of emergency-room revenues."[26]

By 2019, it was clear that during the previous decade the U.S. had spent an excess of $2.1 trillion over what Canada had spent (as a percentage of hospital administrative costs) due to that country's more efficient single payer system.[27] A comparison between the United States and Cuba would have evidenced much greater differences. In 2017, the United States paid private insurers almost $230 billion to manage insurance plans, which meant that the insurers' administrative costs were 19 percent of their outlay. At the same time, Medicare's administrative costs were slightly over 2 percent of what it paid out.[28]

In the United States, 17.8 percent of GDP is devoted to health care while the figure is 11.5 percent in "comparable nations" (meaning rich countries) where people live longer than they do in the United States. Despite the huge sum being spent, many people in the United States either have no health coverage or are under-insured.[29] Ralph Nader notes that, while people in the United States must wade through complex bills from doctors and hospitals, Canadians (who benefit from their provincial health care system) "usually don't even see a bill."[30] However, there is a way that U.S. providers are more skilled than their Canadian counterparts: they learn more about upgrading diagnoses and upcoding levels of service to increase medical reimbursements![31]

UNDER-TREATMENT AND OVER-TREATMENT

Market economies tend to misallocate resources, producing too few of some things (which are not profitable) while producing too many of other things (which are profitable). In medicine, this leads to the simultaneous under-production of some health services and over-production of others. Ironically, both tend to increase the cost of medicine.

People with low incomes in the United States are painfully aware of medical underproduction. When forced to choose between paying for prescriptions or rent, going to the dentist or paying the mortgage, or skipping a medical appointment to buy a car, they feel the stranglehold that the sickness industry has on their lives. An article in *Health Affairs* confirmed that the uninsured are less likely to be treated, resulting in their illnesses progressing and their treatments ultimately becoming more expensive. According to the article's lead author Dr. Andrew Wilper, "they're not getting care that would prevent strokes, heart attacks, amputations and kidney failure."[32] Those without adequate insurance also receive more hurried care when they do get it. They might have little access to office-based care and instead use the Emergency Room, making the ER more crowded for everyone.[33] In Texas, a third of pregnant women go through the first trimester without a single prenatal checkup.[34] This would be an extraordinarily rare occurrence in Cuba, where neighborhood committees, more focused on human costs than the financial aspects of under-treatment, urge necessary prenatal care.

By contrast, there is substantial evidence of over-treatment for those who can afford insurance in the United States. One of the most readable accounts of profit-motivated over-treatment is Stan Cox's *Sick Planet* (2008). He describes how the Parker Hughes Cancer Center in Roseville, Minnesota, went bankrupt after the *Minneapolis Star Tribune* reported that it "had been subjecting cancer patients to excessive testing and treating."[35] When doctors install magnetic resonance imaging (MRI) machines in their offices, they tend to use them 23 percent more than if they have to refer out for a scan. After the purchase price is covered by the first two to three thousand scans, additional ones generate almost pure profit.[36] Over-testing leading to over-treatment is becoming an international trend. A study in Australia confirmed that if "100 patients are each subjected to 10 random diagnostic tests, around 40 of them will be 'found' to have a problem that really isn't there."[37] The pharmaceutical industry has become especially adept at transforming what are serious problems for some into artificial sicknesses. Stan Cox has described how this is done by defining and redefining "a host of medical conditions—erectile dysfunction, female sexual dysfunction, restless legs, sleeplessness, bipolar disorder, attention deficit disorder, social anxiety disorder, and irritable bowel syndrome." What all of these have in common is industry's ability to tele-market their remedies.[38]

Martha Rosenberg has written extensively about the hype over bone-density scans and bone-building drugs as a way to counter osteoporosis, especially in post-menopausal women. She claims that "Bone density machines were dreamed up, placed in doctors' offices and the scans made Medicare reimbursable by Merck to sell its bone drug Fosamax."[39] Fosamax, a prescription medication, is in the category of bisphosphonates. Before the appearance of Fosamax, there were only 750 bone-density machines in medical offices and clinics, but by 1999 eight to ten thousand such machines were in use.[40] Research soon showed both that diet was a major risk factor for fractures (especially with high intake of animal protein) and that bisphosphonates could increase bone brittleness and even increase the risk of fractures.[41] By 2010, the FDA had issued a warning for diseases associated with the use of bisphosphonates.[42]

In a parallel fashion, as more psychiatric drugs were developed, diagnoses of mental illness increased. Between 1987 and 2007, the mental illness disability rate in the United States more than doubled (from one in 184 to one in 76).[43] In the same period, the use of drugs like Ritalin for attention deficit hyperactivity disorder (ADHD) in children (mostly boys) shot up thirty-fold. Though the mental health industry insists on the use of psychoactive drugs, psychiatrist Grace Jackson said in an interview that

There is no evidence that failure to medicate "harms" a psychotic person but there is evidence from neuroimaging studies in humans that old and new antipsychotics contribute to brain tissue loss, especially in the frontal lobes . . . people who were never psychotic or mentally ill can start to experience psychological symptoms upon the withdrawal of these drugs . . .[44]

This means that mental health professionals often misinterpret withdrawal effects as symptoms of the psychosis. A revealing new line of research is the use of "sham surgery" to determine if actual surgery is beneficial. In a 2018 *Scientific American* article, Claudia Wallis explains how, in this kind of trial, patients are randomly assigned either to a group where the surgeon performs the actual surgical procedure or to a group undergoing the first steps of surgery but not the

critical portion.[45] Applying this approach to migraine headache prevention, investigators have demonstrated that sugar pills are effective
for 22 percent of patients, sham acupuncture helps 38 percent, but
sham migraine surgery helps 58 percent.[46] Sham arthroscopic knee
surgery studies indicate that most patients do not benefit from the
procedure. and "would do just as well with physical therapy, weight
loss and exercise."[47] Vertabroplasty, or the mending of fractured verte-
brae by injecting bone cement, became popular during the early 2000s
but sham surgery studies demonstrated that it is no more beneficial
than the placebo procedure.[48] The most startling finding is that for
many patients sham surgery is as effective for blocked arteries as are
angioplasties or stent operations.[49] In a study involving two hundred
patients, physicians carried out either the real procedure or the sham
one. Both groups of patients felt better, had less pain, and improved
on treadmill tests six weeks after surgery. Multiple studies have also
found that stent operations do not reduce the risk of heart attack or
death and that medications with lifestyle changes appear to be the
best treatment for most patients. Nevertheless, over half a million
stent operations and over two million arthroscopic surgeries are done
annually in the world.[50] It is likely that there are many other expensive
but ineffective procedures that are widely used simply to reap profits.

SICKNESS LOOPING

Closely connected to over-treatment is "sickness looping," which
occurs when treatment leads to more sickness and then more treatment. Sickness looping can be traced to (a) treatments applied to
individual patients, (b) the hospital environment, and (c) the medical
system in combination with other sectors of the economy. There is a
plethora of evidence of some individual treatments harming patients
more than helping them. For example, too much radiation can be
unhealthy, despite what the nuclear industry maintains. From 1980 to
2010, the average lifetime dose of non-therapeutic diagnostic radiation increased sevenfold, increasing the risk for cancer. A 2000 study
found that as many as 2 percent of future cancers could be due to CT

scan radiation.[51] Likewise, proton pump inhibitors (PPIs), the second best-selling category of heartburn drugs in 2008, were accounting for $14 billion of sales in the United States. But PPIs appear to be vastly overprescribed for hospitalized patients. Since the drugs inhibit calcium absorption, those taking high-dose PPIs long-term are 2.65 times more likely to have hip fractures. Further, they are twice as likely to develop pneumonia and almost three times as likely to get a potentially deadly infection. Most disturbing, PPIs may actually cause heartburn and acid reflux—the very problems they supposedly treat![52]

Psychiatrists are warned against polypharmacy, or prescribing multiple medications, but they often do so. Research shows that among those taking combinations of Seroquel, Zyprexa, and other antipsychotics, only one of twenty-four experienced worse symptoms when they reduced their intake to a single medication. Since patients often complain that they feel "zonked out" by anti-psychotic drugs, it is not surprising that those receiving a single medication saw at their waist circumferences and triglycerides (fat in the blood) improved, probably due to increased activity. In addition to their questionable efficacy, the extra drugs were contributing to the risk of diabetes and cardiovascular diseases![53]

Martha Rosenberg points out that television advertising in the early 2000s presented hormone replacement therapy (HRT) as an elixir that would prevent diminished memory, loss of sight, and tooth loss. Yet the drugs not only failed to prevent such age-related diseases but actively caused many of them.[54]

To the surprise of many, research subsequently confirmed that HRT "increased the risk of heart attacks by 29%, stroke by 41%, and it doubled the risk of blood clots."[55] A long list of investigations has associated HRT with dementia, shrinking of brain size, hearing loss, gall bladder disease, urinary incontinence, asthma, joint problems, and a variety of cancers. HRT has also been shown to both increase the risk of breast cancer by 26 percent and to make detection more difficult. On top of that, when women quit HRT their rates of breast cancer, ovarian cancer and heart attacks fall. The use of HRT was enormous. By the time it was discredited, sixty-one million prescriptions had been written—enough to treat approximately one third of all women in the United States.[56] What was the response of drug manufacturers to these findings? They waited until the furor died down, changed the phrase "hormone replacement therapy" to "hormone therapy" and restarted marketing "as if nothing had happened."[57]

A second source of sickness looping is the hospital environment itself. According to the Centers for Disease Control (CDC), each year two million Americans contract infectious diseases in hospitals.[58] It has long been known that bringing people with compromised disease resistance into a disease-rich environment is one of the best ways to increase sickness. A recent article by Ralph Nader refers to peer reviewed research from the Johns Hopkins School of Medicine estimating that five thousand deaths result each week from deficiencies in care such as hospital-induced infection, medical malpractice, and inattentiveness. According to Nader, medical analysts believe that "preventable problems in hospitals are the third leading cause of death in America after heart disease and cancer!"[59]

At least as significant a systems problem is the way the sickness industry contributes to illness by generating a wide variety of toxins and accelerating climate change. Doctors' offices and hospitals may evoke images of sterile cleanliness, but medical tools, continuous lights, temperature systems, and unnecessary construction cause enormous amounts of pollution. The pollution, in turn, promotes sickness. Research from Yale University shows that, "If the U.S. health care system were a country, it would rank 13th in the world in terms of greenhouse gas emissions."[60] In 2013, the U.S. health care system caused

significant fractions of national air pollution emissions and impacts, including acid rain (12%), greenhouse gas emissions (10%), smog formation (10%), criteria air pollutants (9%), stratospheric ozone depletion (1%), and carcinogenic and noncarcinogenic air toxics (1–2%). . . . These indirect health burdens are commensurate with the 44,000–98,000 people who die in hospitals each year in the U.S. as a result of preventable medical errors, but are currently not attributed to our health system.[61]

Health care-related emissions are linked to chemically-caused cancers, respiratory disease from air pollutants, ozone depletion, climate change and environmental damage from acid rain. The study's authors estimate total health damages to be 470,000 "disability adjusted life years" (DALYs)—a measure of years lost from sickness, disability, or early death.[62] Ill health from the sickness industry is not constant, but rather increases as the industry expands. Greenhouse emissions from health care grew from 7 percent of the United States' total greenhouse emissions in 2003 to nearly 10 percent in 2013.[63]

The sickness industry also interacts with other sectors of the corporate economy to exacerbate medical problems. Expensive technologies and even the cement for medical buildings contribute to the rapid expansion of a huge variety of extraction industries, which in turn lead to mining and transportation injuries, poisoning of workers and communities, and increased emissions across the world. Obsession with the individual car as the primary mode of transportation was responsible for 4.6 million medically consulted injuries during 2017 (with estimated costs of $433.8 billion) in addition to health effects from extraction and pollution associated with the manufacture of vehicles.[64]

Perhaps most destructive for societal health are antibiotic practices of factory "farms." Over 70% of antibiotics go to livestock, not to people . . . and they are the same drugs needed for urinary tract, intestinal, respiratory, ear, and skin infections in humans. They are also crucial drugs in treating tuberculosis and sexually transmitted diseases.[65]

Massive overuse of antibiotics to fatten animals for slaughter and to compensate for the animals' horribly unsanitary living conditions leads directly to the sale of meat that is contaminated with drug-resistant bacteria. In the United States, seventy thousand people die from antibiotic resistant infections annually and many more become ill.[66]

DRUG LOOPING

Antibiotic resistance is just one way that Big Pharma sticks it to people in the United States. Just as "sickness looping" occurs when treatment loops back on itself and requires more treatment, "drug looping" happens when there are drug "side effects" that lead a physician to prescribe more drugs. For example, anti-psychotics often cause involuntary movements (which can become permanent) requiring treatment with a new set of medications. Some patients refuse an initial drug treatment because they fear a domino effect.

There are big issues with prescribing Ritalin-like drugs (typically stimulants) for children with Attention Deficit Hyperactivity Disorder (ADHD). Between 1987 and 2007, the use of these drugs shot up over thirty-fold. Dr. Leonard Sax explains that a child who does well outside of home and school environments (both of which may expect too much quiet sitting) does not have ADHD. He sees Ritalin-like drugs as academic steroids since they improve the academic performance of most children who take them, but with potentially negative consequences.[67] Two years after Sax's book came out an article was published in *Scientific American* summarizing research that confirmed his hypothesis. There, Gary Stix documented that pharmaceutical companies were pushing ADHD drugs as performance-enhancers. Though they can improve long-term memory, such drugs can also interfere with working memory and complex problem-solving. Other problems include cardiac arrhythmia, seizures, appetite suppression, and sleep disruption.[68]

BIG PHARMA: OVER-DIAGNOSING

Former pharmaceutical representative Gwen Olsen observes that "Children are known to be compliant patients and that makes them a highly desirable market for drugs."[69] Once prodded into taking drugs by their family, school, and psychiatrist, children are likely to dutifully pop prescribed medications and become repeat customers for the drug industry. By 2012, the number of prescriptions for children was rising four times faster than for adults.[70]

Drug manufacturers find artificial ways to generate enthusiasm for their products. When Big Pharma wants to fast-track drug approval, it often flies in patients to hearings so they can testify that a drug deserves to receive a rapid stamp of approval.[71] As mentioned earlier, drug companies often play a central role in the creation and over-diagnosis of "illnesses" whose authenticity is very dubious. People with very real problems are being sold drugs that may not help or could even be worse than traditional approaches. For example, Amgen introduced Prolia in 2010 as a treatment for "post-menopausal women with osteoporosis at high risk of fractures"[72] Prolia received FDA approval even though its results were worse than placebos in some trials. Tests found that patients given Prolia did not do as well as those given Vitamin D and calcium (which are routinely given in bone-drug trials). A study of over sixty-eight thousand patients in the *British Medical Journal* suggests that the bisphosphonate category of drugs—to which Prolia belongs—were of "borderline significance" while Vitamin D plus calcium "significantly reduced the risk of fracture."[73] Furthermore, Prolia has potentially grave side effects, including osteonecrosis of the jaw, atypical fractures, and delayed fracture healing.[74]

In 1997, drug companies established a new beachhead with the legalization of direct-to-consumer (DTC) advertising. Such advertising, usually through the mass media, is directed not at health professionals but rather potential patients. By 2006, Big Pharma was devoting $5.5 billion a year to DTC.[75] Of course, that $5.5 billion was ultimately paid for by those who purchase the products. The advertising led to drugs being used more widely to treat the emotional problems of children or other relatives, especially elderly adults. Within a decade of the initiation of DTC advertising "the number of Americans on antidepressants had doubled to 27 million, or 10% of the population."[76] It was about this time that research began demonstrating that anti-depressants offered little benefit, if any. One of the best-known studies was a 2008 meta-analysis which found that "the new-generation antidepressants do not produce clinically significant improvements in depression in patients who initially have moderate or even very severe depression."[77]

Big Pharma: Overpricing

The U.S. government directly facilitates the profit generation of pharmaceutical giants. With the tremendous clout it has, the U.S. government could insist on lower prices for medications. However, "a legal provision enacted in 2003 prohibited the government from negotiating drug prices for Medicare—a gift of some $50 billion a year or more to the pharmaceutical industry."[78] As huge as this amount is, it pales by comparison to profits from patents. It has taken drug companies centuries to obtain those patents. Fran Quigley writes in *The Nation* that the first known "letters patent" were "issued in 14th-century England to induce foreign craftsmen to relocate there." As the practice expanded, it did not include medicines, considered to be "essential goods." Germany's patent laws specifically excluded medicines in 1877. Patents did not affect medicines in Italy and Sweden until the 1970s and the same was true for Spain until 1992. It was international trade deals such as the GATT and TRIPS that solidified "intellectual property rights" and patents for drugs. Big Pharma argued that such patents were necessary to spark innovation.[79] Nevertheless, the huge discrepancy between the $350 billion in super profits that the industry reaps from patent monopolies and the mere $70 billion it spends on research, tells a different story.[80]

As it is, drug prices are approximately twice as high in the United States as in other wealthy countries.[81] In fact, most drugs are very cheap to manufacture and without patent protection medications "would sell for less than 10 percent of their patent-protected price and often for less than 1 percent," according to Dean Baker.[82] Baker's solution would be government financing of research via direct contracts with companies to develop new drugs, which would then be in the public domain. One effect would be that U.S. Big Pharma "would have much less reason to conceal evidence that drugs are less effective than originally believed or that they could be dangerous under some circumstances."[83] Martha Rosenberg would like to ask Big Pharma, "Why have you raised the price of an insulin vial from $200 to $1,500? Why does Actimmune, for malignant osteoporosis, sell for $350 in Britain and $26,000 in the U.S.?" Comparisons between the United States and other rich countries, however, are only half the story. It is common knowledge that companies sell drugs for much less to poor countries, where people could never afford the prices paid in rich countries. For example, three months' worth of the Hepatitis C drug Sovaldi "sells in India for $900. The list price in the United States is $84,000. This is equivalent to a tariff of more than 40,000 percent."[84]

BIG PHARMA: INTENTIONAL WASTE FOR PROFIT

One of the most fascinating investigations of the enormous over-pricing of drugs is that providers are required to destroy "expired" drugs, despite the Food and Drug Administration's (FDA) being well aware that they are often potent for additional years. The term "expiration date" on drugs merely indicates the point beyond which the FDA will guarantee effectiveness, but many could be effective long after that date. By requiring hospitals and pharmacies to discard "expired" drugs, the FDA is lending a helping hand to Big Pharma.[85]

A hospital in the Boston area had to destroy $200,000 worth of drugs in one year. Pharmacists often take home "expired" drugs for personal use because they are aware of their effectiveness. Many government agencies do the same: for example, the Centers for Disease Control, the Department of Veteran Affairs, and the military all try to save money by using expired drugs (which again demonstrates that the government can be more efficient than the market). In 2016, the Department of Defense alone saved $2.1 billion as part of the Shelf Life Extension Program, which investigates the efficacy of drugs beyond the expiration date.[86] However grateful Big Pharma is for federal and state laws preventing the use of "expired" drugs, the drug makers themselves are quite willing to extend the shelf life of drugs if doing so helps sales and profits in times of shortage!

The safety of most "expired" drugs is now beyond question. The *Journal of Pharmaceutical Sciences* describes research examining 122 medications that found two-thirds of "expired" drugs were stable when a batch was tested. It appears that the average shelf life of these drugs could be extended for four years. The study's authors concluded that safety could be assured by "periodic testing and systematic evaluation" of medications "that have been carefully stored in their sealed container closures."[87] A particularly surprising study appeared in the *Archives of Internal Medicine* concerning medications that had been in a pharmacy for twenty-eight to forty years after their expiration dates. Tests revealed that "12 of 14 medications retained full potency for at least 336 months, and 8 of these for at least 480 months [40 years]" and "Three of these compounds were present at greater than 110% of the labeled content."[88]

Could people be harmed by taking expired medications? When independent news service *ProPublica* spoke with researcher Lee Cantrell, he said that "there has been no recorded instance of such harm in medical literature."[89] As mentioned above, drugs can be tested in batch samples so that those that have lost potency can be identified. How much money is wasted by destruction of good medicines? *ProPublica* estimates that "such squandering eats up about $765 billion a year—as much as a quarter of all the country's health care spending."[90]

The Cuban revolution, during its first decade, directly confronted the "Big Pharma" of its time. Before the revolution, 70 percent of Cuba's pharmaceutical industry was foreign-controlled and only one thousand of four thousand medications in use had therapeutic value. Decree No. 709 (of March 23, 1959) reduced prices of domestic products by 15 percent and imported products by 20 percent. In 1961, the new government nationalized thirty-five warehouses and 370 pharmacies and began shutting down redundant pharmacies. By 1968, urban pharmacies had decreased by more than half, but rural pharmacies had increased fivefold.[91]

SALARIES AND INVESTMENT WEALTH

It's no secret that the U.S. health system lines the pockets of a great many people. Dean Baker points out that the inflated salaries of doctors and dentists in the United States (which are about twice of what they make in other rich countries) leads to an excess cost of about a trillion dollars each decade.[92] This is not only due to general practitioners receiving up to $200,000 per year and specialists' often exceeding $300,000 annually.

It is also because two-thirds of U.S. doctors are specialists, while specialists account for one-third of doctors in most countries. That means that U.S. specialists perform procedures and tests themselves that other lower-paid health care professionals would do elsewhere.[93] In the end, the average U.S. family spends almost $700 annually to keep doctors richer than their counterparts elsewhere.[94]

While Baker provides some of the best data on exposing a range of medical costs, he offers what is probably the worst solution to the high salaries of U.S. professionals. He proposes to bring their salaries down by attracting more doctors from poor countries to practice medicine in the United States. This would be the opposite of Cuba's sending doctors abroad; it would exacerbate the "brain drain" of professionals from these countries and further deprive impoverished people of necessary medical care.[95] A much better approach—short of abolishing capitalism—would be to establish a maximum wage or salary which would be defined as a multiple of the minimum wage. That way the rich could increase their incomes only by proportionally increasing the income of the lowest paid workers.

The true profiteers of the sickness industry are its executives, owners, and investors. *Business Insider* identified the salaries of thirty-one health care executives who were each compensated over $6 million in 2018.[96] In addition to the CEOs of insurance companies, the list included pharmaceutical, equipment, and research executives. The biggest salaries were those of Gilead Sciences CEO John Milligan ($25,961,831), Centene CEO Michael Neidorff ($26,122,414), and Regeneron CEO Lee Schleifer ($26,520,555).[97] Even larger payouts went to the Sackler family, pushers of the addictive pain medication OxyContin. During the first nine months of 2013 "Purdue Pharma paid the family $400 million," and a lawsuit against the Sackler family charges them with having received over $4 billion from Purdue from 2008 to 2016.[98]

The Human Cost of Medicine for Profit

Many of the worst aspects of profit-based medicine do not appear in financial calculations. They include the millions who suffer and die because they cannot afford the care they need and the millions who undergo unnecessary treatment. In 2008, lack of health insurance caused the deaths of 2,200 veterans over the age of sixty-five.[99] A review of pooled data from studies of twenty-six thousand hospitals with thirty-eight million patients found that private for-profit ownership of hospitals is associated with a higher risk of death for patients. The authors noted that for-profit hospitals have extra costs that lead them to skimp on patient care, often by hiring fewer highly skilled personnel.[100] One study of health care plans concluded that "if all 23.7 million American women between ages 50 and 69 years were enrolled in investor-owned, rather than not-for-profit plans, an estimated 5,925 additional breast cancer deaths would be expected."[101]

As Ralph Nader points out, "In Canada, nobody dies due to lack of health insurance."[102] By contrast, when people in the United States realize how much they will have to pay in deductibles, they often put themselves at risk by delaying procedures. For those who do decide to go ahead with a procedure despite not having the resources, they worry about what it will mean. Will they have to declare bankruptcy? Will they have to beg relatives for money? In 2018, one in three of GoFundMe fundraisers were for medical bills. Many delay retirement just to keep their medical insurance. Some even commit crimes, so they can get health care in jail.[103]

Profit-based health care fuels all of this and more. On the one hand, it provides a pernicious incentive for companies to conceal knowledge when drugs are ineffective or cause harm. On the other hand, it fails to develop drugs to cure the diseases prevalent in poor countries. Research published in *The Lancet* found that only twenty-one of the 1,556 new drugs marketed from 1975 to 2004 were for tropical diseases.[104] In fifty years, only one new medicine was introduced to combat tuberculosis, which causes over a million deaths per year. Instead, profit-driven drug research leads to endless quests for sexual performance enhancers and cures for male pattern baldness.[105]

As the pharmaceutical industry continuously invades every aspect of U.S. medicine, bonds between health care providers and patients grow weaker and weaker. I cannot remember the last time I was able to call a doctor's office and get a prescription for a simple problem without getting bogged down in scheduling, waiting, and expensive insurance paperwork. When I do arrive for the appointment, the person performing the critical act of verifying insurance coverage never knows my name. By contrast, in any Cuban city, a person who wants to see a doctor just walks a block or two to the *consultorio*, unless, of course, it's a day scheduled for a home visit. Then the doctor walks to the patient!

Tomorrow's Medicine

In 2009, my wife Barbara Chicherio and I were returning from a Heartwood Forest Council that Jim Scheff had organized at Camp McKee near Kentucky's Red River Gorge, a beautiful area in impoverished Montgomery County. I reminisced of the years we had spent organizing opposition to contamination from incinerators, landfills, manufacturing plants and Monsanto's poisonous chemicals that magically morphed into GMOs. Those struggles bore many similarities to efforts to halt deforestation, which others had organized and we supported. It hit me that they all shared a similar theme: "Stop it!" In virtually all environmental conflicts people demand that capitalists stop whatever they are doing. By the time we arrived in St. Louis, it was clear to me that halting capitalist destruction and creating a better world would require considerably less extraction and manufacture.

For decades, environmental thinkers have written that the best way to reduce toxic contamination is not by "managing" toxins after they are released but by banning their creation, which means reducing a great deal of production. The food industry should be reduced, not by producing less food, but by having food without poisons, artificial preservatives, monocropping, advertising, overpackaging, and control by multinationals. The transportation industry should be reduced, not by making it harder to move around, but by having compact neighborhoods where people can make 80 to 90 percent of their trips by walking or cycling rather than using heavy machines that devote 90 percent of their energy to moving themselves and less than 10 percent to moving people. Home appliances should be reduced, not by eliminating things that people need, but by focusing on production of necessary items designed to last for decades rather than months before falling apart or going out of style. This list could become quite long by including all productive sectors.

One economic sector stood out in my mind that might need expansion in a post-capitalist society: medicine. In 2009, it seemed to me that extending good universal health care throughout the world would require increased production and more energy. However, after my daughter began attending medical school in Cuba, I started reading about the country's health system. A couple of years earlier was when my daughter Rebecca returned from a trip to Mexico and Cuba, called me, and said, "Dad, in Cuba I saw a medical school called ELAM that has students from all over the world and I want to go there to study medicine." After hearing more, I encouraged her to follow her dream and, after taking courses required for beginning medical school, she was off to Havana and I soon visited her there. Reading about its health system, I discovered that Cuba spends vastly less money on medical care than the United States does, while having similar results for life expectancy and infant mortality. That cast doubt upon my earlier idea that medicine would be the only economic area requiring expansion in a post-capitalist society.

As climate catastrophe threatens to end human existence, it becomes increasingly clear that we must tread much, much more lightly on "resources" and vigorously seek to reduce production by focusing less on exchange values and more on use values. But producing what is useful for people rather than increasing profits cannot be the focus of a capitalist society. If Cuba's small economy can improve the health of millions of people across the globe, imagine what could be accomplished if the United States' enormous productive capacity changed from creating useless and destructive junk to producing what people throughout the world actually need!

While many believe that this can be accomplished by focusing on the construction of things, it is actually the emergence and consolidation of a new consciousness that is critical. A post-capitalist United

States would need to nationalize the pharmaceutical industry and stop its extreme waste. Yet Big Pharma's greatest victory has been instilling the belief that life's problems can be solved by taking the right pill. A revolutionary transformation would include the understanding that, though medications can be critical life savers, most remedies should focus on lifestyle changes and ancient and natural healing methods. Curing a drug-dependent society requires that consciousness become a material force in the production of health.

Can Cuba's approach to health care be replicated in the U.S. piecemeal? Some who have been to both countries see a similarity between Urgent Care Centers (UCCs) and polyclinics. Though both provide quick treatment, UCCs do not have a geographically designed service area and preserve the core corporate structures of medicine. The beginning point of a new health care system is a fundamental change in the relationship between healers and patients. Efforts to do so in a corporate-controlled industry is like trying to swim upstream from the bottom of Niagara Falls. Nevertheless, large numbers of professionals recognize the calamity of U.S. medicine and many strike out on their own.

A notable effort to apply the Cuban approach to medicine in the United States is the Birthing Project U.S.A. (BPUSA). The Birthing Project was the first community-based birthing program for African Americans in the United States. According to Kathryn Hall-Trujillo, who founded the program in 1998, "It trains people to work with pregnant women and to connect with them through the first year of the life of the infant."[106]

The Birthing Project aims for intervention at critical periods to improve birth outcomes, giving great importance to the mother's health when she becomes pregnant. By 2019, BPUSA had been replicated over seventy times in the U.S., Canada, and Honduras.[107]

Hall-Trujillo is grateful for the BPUSA's partnership with Cuba and the support that many ELAM students have given: "We are a coming home place for ELAM students—they see working with us as a way to put into practice what they learned at ELAM. Many students cannot afford the debt of going to medical school in the United States and we encourage students to think about going to ELAM."[108] BPUSA's medical director is Dr. Sarpoma Sefa-Boakye, a graduate of ELAM, who coordinates obtaining supplies and makes sure that the program's clients know how to get medical services. Studying at ELAM greatly aided her in performing medical tasks because

> [BPUSA] is very hands on with a community approach. It focuses on community development by encouraging each group to solve its own problems with assistance from the medical system . . . medical staff look at the issues that are important for a community [including] the number of children per family and what type of support they need for pediatric problems.[109]

Sefa-Boakye also feels that ELAM helped prepare her for her current duties at BPUSA because the project focuses on the most needy populations and emphasizes the role of women as mentors.[110] This contrasts sharply with U.S. medical schools where training focuses on sophisticated procedures rather than teaching patients to incorporate the knowledge that already exists in their communities.

There are large numbers of healers in the United States who are not hooked up with money-making corporations, and there are thousands upon thousands of individuals working to change the health system so that it benefits people rather than corporate investors. With the medical establishment showing so little willingness to change, are all such efforts in vain? It is important to remember that there were divisions among Cuban doctors and students during the decade that preceded the revolution. Those who demanded that medical care be extended to poor, black, and rural Cuba later became the foundation of the continuously changing system that began in 1959 based on their dreams.

Today, an island with a very small percentage of the world's population may be showing humanity how it can confront not only medical, but a host of environmental and social problems as it simultaneously recreates medicine and produces less of what is not needed. Its revolutionaries had a dream. It is the task of everyone hoping for a better global medicine to keep that dream alive.

HOW CHE GUEVARA TAUGHT CUBA TO CONFRONT COVID-19

Beginning in December 1951, Ernesto "Che" Guevara took a nine-month break from medical school to travel by motorcycle through Argentina, Chile, Peru, Colombia, and Venezuela. One of his goals was gaining practical experience with leprosy. On the night of his twenty-fourth birthday, Che was at La Colonia de San Pablo in Peru where he swam across the river to join the lepers. He walked among six hundred lepers, living in jungle huts, looking after themselves in their own way.

Che would not have been satisfied to just study and sympathize with lepers. He wanted to be with them and understand their existence. Che's contact with people who were poor and hungry at the same time they were sick transformed him. He envisioned a new medicine with doctors who would serve the greatest number of people with preventive care and public awareness of hygiene. A few years later, Che joined Fidel Castro's July 26th Movement as a doctor and was among the eighty-one men aboard the *Granma* as it landed in Cuba on December 2, 1956.

Revolutionary Medicine

After the January 1, 1959, victory, the new Cuban Constitution included Che's dream of free medical-care-for-all as a human right. An understanding of the failings of disconnected social systems led the revolutionary government to build hospitals and clinics in underserved parts of the island at the same time it began addressing crises of literacy, racism, poverty, and housing. Cuba overhauled its clinics in 1964 and again in 1974 to better link communities and patients. By 1984, Cuba had introduced doctor-nurse teams who lived in the neighborhoods where they had offices (*consultorios).*

As the United States became ever more bellicose Cubans organized the Committees for Defense of the Revolution (CDRs) in 1960 to defend the country. The CDRs also prepared to move the elderly, disabled, sick, and mentally ill to higher ground if a hurricane approached, thus intertwining health care and foreign affairs, a connection that has been maintained throughout Cuba's history.

Cuba's medical revolution was based on extending medical care beyond the major cities and into the rural communities that needed it most, so it was a short step to extend that assistance to other nations. The revolutionary government sent doctors to Chile after a 1960 earthquake and a medical brigade in 1963 to Algeria, which was fighting for independence from France. These set the stage for the country's international programs of medical aid, which grew during the decades and now includes the COVID-19 pandemic.

In the late 1980s and early 1990s, two disasters threatened the very existence of the country. The first victim of AIDS died in 1986. In December 1991, the Soviet Union collapsed, ending its $5 billion annual subsidy, disrupting international commerce and sending the Cuban economy into a free fall that exacerbated AIDS problems. A perfect storm for AIDS infection appeared on the horizon. The HIV infection rate for the Caribbean region was second only to southern Africa, where a third of a million Cubans had recently been during the Angolan wars. The embargo reduced the availability of drugs (including those for HIV/AIDS), made existing pharmaceuticals out-rageously expensive, and disrupted the financial infrastructure used for drug purchases. Desperately needing funds, Cuba opened the floodgate of tourism, bringing an increase in sex being exchanged for money .

The government drastically reduced services in all areas except two: education and health care. Its research institutes developed Cuba's own diagnostic HIV test by 1987, and more than 12 million tests were completed by 1993. By 1990, when homosexuals had become the island's primary HIV victims, anti-gay prejudice was officially challenged as schools taught that homosexuality was a fact of life. Condoms were provided free at doctors' offices. Despite the expense, Cuba provided antiretroviral drugs free to patients.

Cuba's united and well-planned effort to cope with HIV/AIDS paid off. At the same time Cuba had 200 AIDS cases, New York City (with about the same population) had 43,000 cases. Despite having a small fraction of the wealth and resources of the United States, Cuba had overcome the devastating effects of the US blockade and had imple-mented an AIDS program superior to that of the country seeking to destroy it. During this "Special Period," Cubans experienced longer lives and lower infant mortality rates in comparison to the United States. Cuba had inspired healers throughout the world to believe that a country with a coherent and caring medical system can thrive, even against tremendous odds.

COVID-19 HITS CUBA

Overcoming the HIV/AIDS and Special Period crises prepared Cuba for COVID-19. Aware of the intensity of the pandemic, Cuba knew that it had two inseparable tasks: first, it must take care of its own with a comprehensive program, and, second, it must share its capabilities internationally.

The government immediately addressed a crucial shortage—it altered the equipment of nationalized factories (which usually made school uniforms) to manufacture medical masks. Though this proved very difficult in a market-driven economy it provided an ample supply for Cuba by the middle of April 2020, when the United States, with its enormous productive capacity, was still suffering a shortage.

Discussions at the highest levels of the Cuban Ministry of Public Health (MINSAP) prepared the national policy. There would need to be massive testing to determine who had been infected. Infected persons would need to be quarantined, while, at the same time they had to have adequate food and other necessities. Contact tracing would be used to determine who else might be exposed. Medical staff would need to go door-to-door to check on the health of every citizen. *Consultorio* (doctor office) staff would give special attention to everyone in the neighborhood who might be at high risk.

By March 2, Cuba had instituted the Novel Coronavirus Plan for Prevention and Control.[1] Within four days, it expanded the plan to include taking the temperature of and possibly isolating infected incoming travelers. These occurred before Cuba's first confirmed COVID-19 diagnosis on March 11. Cuba had its first confirmed COVID-19 fatality by March 22, when there were thirty-five confirmed cases, almost 1,000 patients under observation in hospitals, and over 30,000 people under surveillance at home. The next day it banned the entry of non-resident foreigners, which took a deep bite out of the country's tourism revenue.[2]

That was the day that Cuba's Civil Defense went on alert to respond rapidly to COVID-19 and the Havana Defense Council decided that there was a serious problem in the city's Vedado district. The district is famed for being the largest home for foreign visitors who stay longer than tourists and were more likely to have been exposed to the virus. By April 3, the district was closed. As Merriam Ansara witnessed, "Anyone with a need to enter or leave must prove that they have been tested and are free of COVID-19." The Civil Defense made sure stores were supplied and that all vulnerable people received regular medical checks.[3] Vedado had eight confirmed cases, a lot for a small area. Cuban health officials wanted the virus to remain at the "local spread" stage, when it can be traced as it goes from one person to another. They sought to prevent it from entering the "community spread" stage when tracing is not possible because it is moving out of control. Cuba had enough test kits to trace contacts of persons who had contracted the virus, while at the same time US health professionals were complaining of insufficient personal protective equipment (PPE) and testing was so sparse that contacts of infected patients had to *ask* to be tested (rather than health workers testing contacts of infected patients).

Also during late March and early April 2020, Cuban hospitals were changing work patterns to minimize contagion. Havana doctors went into Salvador Allende Hospital for fifteen days, staying overnight within an area designated for medical staff. Then they moved to an area separate from patients where they lived for another fifteen days and were tested before returning home. They stayed at home without leaving for another fifteen days and were tested before resuming practice. This 45-day period of isolation prevented medical staff from bringing disease to the community by daily back-and-forth trips to work.

The medical system in Cuba extends from the *consultorio* to every family. Third-, fourth-, and fifth-year medical students are assigned by *consultorio* doctors to go to specific homes each day. Their tasks include obtaining survey data from residents or making extra visits to the elderly, infants, and those with respiratory problems. These visits gather preventive medicine data that is used by those in the highest decision-making positions of the country. When students bring their data, doctors use a red pen to mark "hot spots" where extra care is necessary. Neighborhood doctors meet regularly at clinics to talk about what each doctor is doing, what they are discovering, what new procedures the Cuban Ministry of Public Health is adopting, and how the intense work is affecting medical staff.

In this way, every Cuban citizen and every health care worker, from those at neighborhood doctors' offices through those at the most esteemed research institutes, has a part in determining health policy. Cuba currently has 89,000 doctors, 84,000 nurses, and 9,000 students scheduled to graduate from medical studies in 2020. The Cuban people would not tolerate the head of the country ignoring medical advice, spouting nonsensical statements, and determining policy based on what would be most profitable for corporations.

The Cuban government approved free distribution of the homeo-pathic medicine PrevengHo-Vir to residents of Havana and Pinar del Rio province.[4] Susana Hurlich was one of many receiving it. On April 8, 2020, Dr. Yaisen, one of three doctors at the *consultorio* two blocks from her home came to the door with a small bottle of PrevengHo-Vir and told her how to use it. Instructions warn that it reinforces the immune system, but is not a substitute for Interferon Alpha 2B and is not a vaccine. Hurlich believes that something important "about Cuba's medical system is that rather than being two-tiered, as is often the case in other countries, with 'classical medicine' on the one hand and 'alternative medicine' on the other, Cuba has ONE health system that includes it all. When you study to become a doctor, you also learn about homeopathic medicine in all its forms."[5]

Global Solidarity in the Time of COVID-19

A powerful model. Perhaps the most critical component of Cuba's medical internationalism during COVID-19 has been creating an example of how a country can confront the disease with a compas-sionate and competent plan. Public health officials around the world were inspired by Cuba's actions.

Transfer of knowledge. When viruses that cause Ebola virus dis-ease, which are mainly in sub-Saharan Africa, increased dramatically in fall 2014, much of the world panicked. Soon, over 20,000 people were infected, more than 8,000 had died, and worries mounted that the death toll could reach into hundreds of thousands. The United States provided military support; other countries promised money. Cuba was the first nation to respond with what was most needed: sending 103 nurse and 62 doctor volunteers to Sierra Leone. Then it did something even more important to fight Ebola: Cuba trained volunteers from other nations at Havana's Pedro Kourí Institute of Tropical Medicine. In total, Cuba taught 13,000 Africans, 66,000 Latin Americans, and 620 Caribbeans how to treat Ebola without themselves becoming infected. Sharing understanding on how to organize a health system is the highest level of knowledge a country can transfer.

Venezuela has attempted to replicate fundamental aspects of the Cuban health model on a national level, and this has served Venezuela well in combating COVID-19. In 2018, residents of Altos de Lidice organized seven communal councils, including one for community health. A resident made space in his home available to the Communal Healthcare System initiative so that a Cuban doctor could have an office. Dr. Gutierrez now coordinates data collections to identify at-risk residents and visits all residents at home to explain how to avoid infection by COVID-19. Nurse del Valle Marquez is a Chavista who helped implement the Barrio Adentro when the first Cuban doctors arrived. She remembers that residents had never seen a doctor inside their community, but when the Cubans arrived "we opened our doors to the doctors, they lived with us, they ate with us, and they worked among us."[6]

Stories like this permeate Venezuela. As a result of building a Cuban-type system, *Telesur* reported that by April 11, 2020, the Venezuelan government had conducted 181,335 early Polymerase Chain Reaction (PCR) tests in time to have the lowest infection rate in Latin America. Venezuela had only six infections per million citizens, whereas neighboring Brazil had 104 infections per million.[7]

When Rafael Correa was president of Ecuador, over 1,000 Cuban doctors formed the backbone of its health care system. Lenin Moreno was elected in 2017 and Cuban doctors were soon expelled, leaving public medicine in chaos. Moreno followed recommendations of the International Monetary Fund to slash Ecuador's health budget by 36 percent, leaving it without health care professionals, without PPE, and, above all, without a coherent health care system. At the same time Venezuela and Cuba had 27 COVID-19 deaths, Ecuador's largest city, Guayaquil, had an estimated death toll of 7,600.[8]

International medical response. Cuban medicine is perhaps best known for its internationalism. A clear example is the devastating earthquake that pounded Haiti in 2010. Cuba sent medical staff who lived among Haitians and stayed months or even years after the earth-quake. U.S. doctors did not sleep where Haitian victims huddled, returned to luxury hotels at night, and departed after a few weeks. John Kirk coined the term "disaster tourism" to describe the way that many rich countries respond to medical crises in poor countries.

The commitment that Cuban medical staff show internationally is a continuation of the effort that the country made over three decades to find the best way to strengthen bonds between caregiving profession-als and those they serve. By 2008, Cuba had sent over 120,000 health care professionals to 154 countries; its doctors had cared for over 70 million people in the world; and almost 2 million people owed their lives to Cuban medical services.

The Associated Press reported that when COVID-19 went world-wide, Cuba had 37,000 medical workers in 67 countries. It soon deployed additional doctors to Suriname, Jamaica, Dominica, Belize, Saint Vincent and the Grenadines, St. Kitts and Nevis, Venezuela, and Nicaragua.[9] On April 16, *Granma* reported that "21 brigades of health care professionals have been deployed to join national and local efforts in 20 countries."[10] The same day, Cuba sent two hundred health personnel to Qatar.[11]

As northern Italy became the epicenter of COVID-19 cases, one of its hardest hit cities was Crema in the Lombardy region. The emer-gency room at the only hospital was filled to capacity. On March 26, Cuba sent fifty-two doctors and nurses who set up a field hospital with three ICU beds and thirty-two other beds with oxygen. A smaller and poorer Caribbean nation was one of the few aiding a major European power. Cuba's intervention took its toll. By April 17, thirty of its medi-cal professionals who went abroad tested positive for COVID-19.[12]

Bringing the world to Cuba. The flip side of Cuba's sending medical staff across the globe is the people it has brought to the island, both students and patients. When Cuban doctors were in the Republic of the Congo in 1966, they saw students studying independently under streetlights at night and arranged for them to come to Havana. They brought in even more African students during the Angolan wars of

1975–1988 and then brought large numbers of Latin American students to study medicine following Hurricanes Mitch and Georges. The number of students coming to Cuba to study expanded even more in 1999 when it opened classes at the Latin American School of Medicine (ELAM). By 2020, ELAM had trained 30,000 doctors from over a hundred countries.

Cuba also has a history of bringing foreign patients for treatment. After the 1986 nuclear meltdown at Chernobyl, 25,000 patients, mostly children, came to the island for treatment, with some staying for months or years. Cuba opened its doors, hospital beds, and a youth summer camp.

Thus, the March 18 events regarding the British cruise ship MS *Braemar* is consistent with a pattern. On March 12, nearly fifty crew members and passengers either had COVID-19 or were showing symptoms as the ship approached the Bahamas, a British Commonwealth nation. Since the *Braemar* flew the Bahamian flag as a Commonwealth vessel, there should have been no problem disembarking those aboard for treatment and return to the United Kingdom. But the Bahamian Ministry of Transport declared that the cruise ship would "not be permitted to dock at any port in the Bahamas and no persons will be permitted to disembark the vessel."[13] During the next five days, the United States, Barbados (another Commonwealth nation), and several other Caribbean countries turned it away. On March 18, Cuba became the only country to allow the *Braemar*'s over 1,000 crew members and passengers to dock. Treatment at Cuban hospitals was offered to those who felt too sick to fly. Most went by bus to José Martí International Airport for flights back to the United Kingdom. Before leaving, *Braemar* crew members displayed a banner reading "I love you Cuba!"[14] Passenger Anthea Guthrie posted on her Facebook page: "They have made us not only feel tolerated, but actually welcome."[15]

Medicine for all. In 1981, there was a particularly bad outbreak of the mosquito-borne dengue fever in Cuba, which hits the island every few years. At this time, many first learned of the very high level of Cuba's research institutes, which had created Interferon Alpha 2B to success-fully treat dengue. As Helen Yaffe points out, "Cuba's interferon has shown its efficacy and safety in the therapy of viral diseases including Hepatitis B and C, shingles, HIV-AIDS, and dengue."[16] It accom-plished this by preventing complications that could worsen a patient's condition and result in death. The efficacy of the drug survived for decades, and, in 2020, it became vitally important as a potential cure for COVID-19. What also survived was Cuba's eagerness to develop a multiplicity of drugs and share them with other nations.

Cuba has sought to work cooperatively toward drug development with countries such as China, Venezuela, and Brazil. Collaboration with Brazil resulted in meningitis vaccines at a cost of 95 cents rather than $15 to $20 per dose. Finally, Cuba teaches other countries to produce medications themselves so they do not have to rely on pur-chasing them from rich countries.

In order to effectively cope with disease, drugs are frequently sought for three goals: *tests* to determine those who are infected; *treatments* to help ward off or cure problems, and *vaccines* to prevent infections. As soon as PRC rapid tests were available (tests that are highly sensi-tive and specific that yield quick and accurate results), Cuba began using them widely throughout the island. Cuba developed both Interferon Alpha 2B (a recombinant protein) and PrevengHo-Vir (a homeopathic medication). *Telesur* reported that by April 20, over 45 countries had requested Cuba's Inteferon in order to control and then get rid of the virus.[17]

Cuba's Center for Genetic Engineering and Biotechnology (CIGB) is seeking to create a vaccine against COVID-19. CIGB Director of Biomedical Research, Dr. Gerardo Guillén, confirmed that his team is collaborating with Chinese researchers in Yongzhou, Hunan prov-ince, to create a vaccine to stimulate the immune system, one that can be taken through the nose, which is the route of COVID-19 trans-mission. Whatever Cuba develops, it is certain that it will be shared with other countries at low cost, unlike US medications, which are patented at taxpayer expense so that private pharmaceutical giants can price-gouge those who need the medication.

Countries that have not learned how to share. Cuban solidarity missions show a genuine concern that often seems to be lacking in health care providers from other countries. Medical associations in Venezuela, Brazil, and other countries are often hostile to Cuban doctors. Yet they cannot find enough of their own doctors to go to dangerous communities or travel to rural areas by donkey or canoe as Cuban doctors do.

When in Peru in 2010, I visited the Pisco *policlínico*. Its Cuban director, Leopoldo García Mejías, explained that then-president Alan García did not want additional Cuban doctors and that they had to keep quiet in order to remain in Peru. Cuba is well aware that it has to adjust each medical mission to adapt to the political climate.

There is at least one exception to Cuban doctors remaining in a country according to the whims of the political leadership. Cuba began providing medical attention in Honduras in 1998. During the first eighteen months of Cuba's efforts in Honduras, the infant mortality dropped from 80.3 to 30.9 deaths per 1,000 live births. Political moods changed, and, in 2005, Honduran health minister Merlin Fernández decided to kick Cuban doctors out. However, this led to so much opposition that the government changed its course and allowed the Cubans to stay.

There is a noteworthy disaster when a country refused an offer of Cuban aid. After the 2005 Hurricane Katrina, 1,586 Cuban health care professionals were prepared to go to New Orleans. President George W. Bush rejected the offer, acting as if it would be better for American citizens to die than to admit the quality of Cuban aid.

Though the US government does not take kindly to students attending ELAM, they are still able to apply what they learn when they come home. In 1988, Kathryn Hall-Trujillo of Albuquerque, New Mexico, founded the Birthing Project USA (BPUSA), which trains advocates to work with African-American women and connect with them through the first year of the infant's life. She is grateful for BPUSA's partnership with Cuba and the support that many ELAM students have given. In 2018, she told me "We are a coming home place for ELAM students—they see working with us as a way to put into practice what they learned at ELAM."

Cuban doctor Julio López Benítez recalled to me in 2017 that when the country revamped its clinics in 1974 the old clinic model meant patients going to clinics but the new model was clinics going to patients. Similarly, as ELAM graduate Dr. Melissa Barber looked at her South Bronx neighborhood during COVID-19, she realized that though most of the United States told people to go to public health agencies, what people need is a community approach that recruits trained organizers to go to the people. Dr. Barber is working in a coalition with South Bronx Unite, the Mott Haven Mamas, and many local tenant associations. As in Cuba, they are trying to identify those in the community who are vulnerable, including "the elderly, people who have infants and small children, homebound people, people that have multiple morbidities and are really susceptible to a virus like this one."[18]

At the same time members of the coalition discover who needs help, they seek resources such as groceries, PPE, medications, and treatment. In short, the approach of the South Bronx coalition is going to homes to ensure that people do not fall through the cracks. In contrast, the US national policy is for each state and each municipality to do what it feels like doing, which means that instead of having a few cracks that a few people fall through, there are enormous chasms with large groups careening into them. What countries with market economies need are actions like those in the South Bronx and Cuba, carried out on a national scale.

This was what Che Guevara envisioned in 1951. Decades before COVID-19 jumped from person to person, Che's imagination went from doctor to doctor. Or perhaps many shared their own visions so widely that after 1959 Cuba brought revolutionary medicine anywhere it could. Obviously, Che did not design the intricate organization of Cuba's current medical system. But he was followed by healers who wove additional designs into a fabric that now unfolds across continents. At certain times in history, thousands or millions of people see similar images of a different future. If their ideas spread broadly enough during the hour that social structures are disintegrating, then a revolutionary idea can become a material force in building a new world.

NOTES

Preface

1. Ian Angus, *Facing the Anthropocene* (New York: Monthly Review Press, 2016), 20.
2. Ross Danielson, *Cuban Medicine* (New Brunswick, NJ: Transaction Books, 1979), 158, 171.
3. Michael A. Lebowitz. *The Contradictions of Real Socialism.* (New York: Monthly Review Press, 2012), 12.
4. Here and in what follows "Zaire" will be used consistently if sometimes anachronistically to refer to the former Belgian Congo, which today is the Democratic Republic of Congo. "The Congo" will be used to refer to its neighbor, the former French colony that is today Republic of Congo.

1. The Three Thousand Who Stayed

1. Ross Danielson, *Cuban Medicine* (New Brunswick, NJ: Transaction, 1979), 22.
2. Ibid., 221–22.
3. José R. Ruíz Hernández, *Cuba, Revolución Social y Salud Pública (1959–1984)* (Havana: Editorial Ciencias Médicas 2008), 13; Danielson, *Cuban Medicine*, 131–33, 222–24.
4. Julia E. Sweig, *Cuba: What Everyone Needs to Know* (Oxford: Oxford University Press, 2009), 37; Danielson, *Cuban Medicine*, 103–4.
5. Ibid., 107.
6. There does not seem to be any connection with the national political

party, Ortodoxos, which attracted a young Fidel Castro in 1947. See Peter G. Bourne, *Fidel* (New York: Dodd, Mead,1986), 39, 53.

7. Ruíz, *Cuba, Revolución Social y Salud Pública*, 10.
8. Ibid., 17.
9. Berta L. Castro Pacheco et al., *Cuban Experience in Child Health Care: 1959–2006* (Havana: Ministry of Public Health, 2010), 5.
10. Candace Wolf, "The Zen of Healing: Spoken Histories of Dr. José Gilberto Fleites Batista and Dr. Gilberto Fleites Gonzalez," Havana, Cuba, January 2013, unpublished manuscript. Dr. José Gilberto Fleites Batista was born in 1925.
11. Author's interview with Dr. Julio López Benítez (born 1933), Havana, Cuba, December 26, 2013.
12. Roberto E. Capote Mir, "La evolución de los servicios de salud y la estructura socioeconómica en Cuba, Segundo Parte: Periódo posrevolucionario" (Havana: Instituto de Desarollo de la Salud, 1979), 53; Ruíz, *Cuba, Revolución Social y Salud Pública*, 29.
13. Ruíz, *Cuba, Revolución Social y Salud Pública*, 43–44, 64.
14. Author's interview with Dr. Enzo Dueñas Gómez (born 1929), Havana, Cuba, December 26, 2013.
15. Author's interview with Dr. Felipe Cárdenas Gonzáles (born 1935), Havana, Cuba, December 26, 2013.
16. Danielson, *Cuban Medicine*, 141.
17. Author's interviews with Dr. Oscar Mena Hector (born 1951), December 21, 2013, and January 1, 2014.
18. Wolf, "The Zen of Healing."
19. Hedelberto López Blanch, *Historias Secretas de Médicos Cubanos* (Havana: Centro Cultural de la Torriente Brau, 2005). Dr. Sara Perelló Perelló was born in 1920. Dr. Pablo Risk Habib was born in 1930. Dr. Zoila Italia Suárez was born in1927.
20. López Blanch, *Historias Secretas*, 9, 216.
21. Ibid., 223.
22. Ibid., 217–18.
23. Ibid., 235.
24. Ibid., 236.
25. Ibid., 224.
26. Ibid., 221.
27. Danielson, *Cuban Medicine*, 120.
28. Capote, "La evolución de los servicios de salud," 57.
29. Danielson, *Cuban Medicine*, 134.
30. Karl Marx, *The Critique of Hegel's Philosophy of Right*, cited in Georg Lukács, *History and Class Consciousness* (Cambridge, MA: MIT Press, 1968), 2.

31. Linda M. Whiteford and Lawrence G. Branch, *Primary Health Care in Cuba: The Other Revolution* (Lanham, MD: Rowman and Littlefield, 2008), 20.

32. Ibid., 54; Castro Pacheco, *Cuban Experience in Child Health Care: 1959–2006*, 42.

2. Birth of the Cuban Polyclinic

1. See chapter 1.

2. Ross Danielson, *Cuban Medicine* (New Brunswick, NJ: Transaction, 1979).

3. John M. Kirk and Michael H. Erisman, *Cuban Medical Internationalism: Origins, Evolution and Goals* (New York: Palgrave Macmillan, 2009); Linda M. Whiteford and Lawrence G. Branch, *Primary Health Care in Cuba: The Other Revolution* (Lanham, MD: Rowman and Littlefield, 2008); Candace Wolf, "The Zen of Healing: Two Surgeons Speak, Spoken Histories of Dr. José Gilberto Fleites Batista and Dr. Gilberto Fleites Gonzalez," Havana, January 2013 (unpublished manuscript).

4. José R. Ruíz Hernández, *Cuba, Revolución Social y Salud Pública 1959⊠1984* (Havana: Editorial Ciencias Médicas, 2008).

5. Danielson, *Cuban Medicine*, 163, 180.

6. Whiteford and Branch, *Primary Health Care in Cuba*, 20.

7. Vicente Navarro, "Health, Health Services, and Health Planning in Cuba," *International Journal of Health Services* 2/3 (1972), 410.

8. Ibid., 426.

9. Ruíz, *Cuba, Revolución Social y Salud Pública*, 88.

10. Danielson, *Cuban Medicine*, 170.

11. Ruíz, *Cuba, Revolución Social y Salud Pública*, 61.

12. Navarro, "Health Planning in Cuba," 414.

13. Ibid., 415.

14. Ibid., "Health Planning in Cuba," 414.

15. Danielson, *Cuban Medicine*, 143.

16. Navarro, "Health Planning in Cuba," 412.

17. Ibid., 411; Danielson, *Cuban Medicine*, 164.

18. Ruíz, *Cuba, Revolución Social y Salud Pública*, 11.

19. Julia E. Sweig, *Cuba: What Everyone Needs to Know* (New York: Oxford University Press, 2009), 45.

20. Danielson, *Cuban Medicine*, 153.

21. Ibid., 178.

22. Roberto E. Capote Mir, *La Evolución de los Servicios de Salud y la Estructura Socioeconómica en Cuba, 2a Parte: Periódo Posrevolucionario* (Havana: Instituto de Desarollo de la Salud, 1979), 41; Ruíz, *Cuba, Revolución Social y Salud Pública*, 48; Danielson, *Cuban Medicine*, 164.

23. Ruíz, *Cuba, Revolución Social y Salud Pública*, 29.
24. Ibid., 62.
25. Danielson, *Cuban Medicine*, 166–67.
26. Ruíz, *Cuba, Revolución Social y Salud Pública*, 43, 56–57.
27. Dr. María Luísa Lima Beltrán, interview with the author, Havana, December 23, 2013.
28. Ibid.
29. Danielson, *Cuban Medicine*, 169.
30. Navarro, "Health Planning in Cuba," 424.
31. Dr. Oscar Mena Hector, interview with the author, Havana, December 21, 2013, and January 1, 2014.
32. Ibid.
33. Navarro, "Health Planning in Cuba," 409.
34. Ibid., 408.
35. Ibid., 428.
36. Danielson, *Cuban Medicine*, 147.
37. Ruíz, *Cuba, Revolución Social y Salud Pública*, 40.
38. Ibid., 59–60.
39. Ibid., 52–53.
40. Danielson, *Cuban Medicine*, 171.
41. Navarro, "Health Planning in Cuba," 424; Danielson, *Cuban Medicine*, 173.
42. Danielson, *Cuban Medicine*, 172–73.
43. Ibid., 173.
44. Ibid., 175.
45. Navarro, "Health Planning in Cuba," 408.
46. Ibid., 424.
47. Danielson, *Cuban Medicine*, 171.
48. Navarro, "Health Planning in Cuba," 431.
49. Berta L. Castro Pacheco et al., *Cuban Experience in Child Health Care: 1959–2006* (Havana: Ministry of Public Health, 2010).
50. Whiteford and Branch, *Primary Health Care in Cuba*, 54.
51. Navarro, "Health Planning in Cuba," 403.
52. Danielson, *Cuban Medicine*, 144.
53. Hedelberto López Blanch, *Historias Secretas de Médicos Cubanos* (Havana: Centro Cultural de la Torriente Brau, 2005), 4.
54. Navarro, "Health Planning in Cuba," 429.
55. Dr. Felipe Cárdenas Gonzáles, interview with the author, Havana, December 26, 2013.
56. Dr. Enzo Dueñas Gómez, interview with the author, Havana, December 26, 2013.
57. Cárdenas, interview with the author.

58. Navarro, "Health Planning in Cuba," 414.
59. Ibid., 413.
60. Ibid., 419.
61. Dr. María Luísa Lima, interview with the author.
62. Peter G. Bourne, *Fidel: A Biography of Fidel Castro* (New York: Dodd, Mead, 1986), 196.
63. Hedelberto López Blanch, interview with the author, Havana, January 10, 2017.
64. Sweig, *Cuba*, 48.
65. Navarro, "Health Planning in Cuba," 414.
66. Ruíz, *Cuba, Revolución Social y Salud Pública*, 88.
67. Dr C. Francisco Rojas Ochoa, "The Number of Physicians in Cuba 1959–1968," *Revista Cubana de Salud Pública* 41/1 (2015): 147–51.
68. Navarro, "Health Planning in Cuba," 414, 419.

3. Cuba's First Military Doctors

1. Piero Gleijeses, *Conflicting Missions: Havana, Washington, and Africa, 1959–1976* (Chapel Hill: University of North Carolina Press, 2002), 61.
2. Ibid., 22.
3. Peter G. Bourne, *Fidel: A Biography of Fidel Castro* (New York: Dodd, Mead, 1986), 255.
4. Gleijeses, *Conflicting Missions*, 30, 60, 61.
5. Bourne, *Fidel*, 260; Gleijeses, *Conflicting Missions*, 80, 85.
6. Gleijeses, *Conflicting Missions*, 87.
7. Ibid., 111, 114.
8. Bourne, *Fidel*, 261.
9. Ibid., 260.
10. Piero Gleijeses, "Jorge Risquet," in *Encyclopedia of African American Culture and History: The Black Experience in the Americas*, ed. Colin A. Palmer (New York: Macmillan, 2006).
11. Gleijeses, *Conflicting Missions*, 161, 163, 170, 171.
12. Ibid., 183.
13. Ibid., 185.
14. Hedelberto López Blanch, *Historias Secretas de Médicos Cubanos* (Havana: Centro Cultural de la Torriente Brau, 2005), 113, 114.
15. Gleijeses, *Conflicting Missions*, 187.
16. Ibid., 190–91.
17. Ibid., 191, 208.
18. Ibid., 183–84; Dr. Juan Antonio Sánchez, interview by Don Fitz, February 9, 2016, Havana.
19. Gleijeses, *Conflicting Missions*, 71, 73.
20. Ibid., 89, 188, 208.

21. López Blanch, *Historias Secretas*, 67, 89.

22. Ibid., 76–77.

23. Ibid.

24. Gleijeses, *Conflicting Missions*, 136, 166.

25. Dr. Rodolfo Puente Ferro, interview by López Blanch, *Historias Secretas*, 101.

26. Gleijeses, *Conflicting Missions*, 199; Dr. Domingo Díaz Delgado, interview by López Blanch, *Historias Secretas*, 115.

27. Dr. Rafaél Zerquera Palacios, interview by López Blanch, *Historias Secretas*, 25.

28. Dr. Diego Lagomasino Comesaña, interview by López Blanch, *Historias Secretas*, 60.

29. Dr. Héctor Vera Acosta, interview by López Blanch, *Historias Secretas*, 53.

30. Dr. Rodrigo Álvarez Cambras, interview by López Blanch, *Historias Secretas*, 75.

31. Dr. Diego Lagomasino Comesaña, interview by López Blanch, *Historias Secretas*, 56–57.

32. Dr. Rafaél Zerquera Palacios, interview by López Blanch, *Historias Secretas*, 22–23.

33. Gleijeses, *Conflicting Missions*, 154, 200.

34. Dr. Rafaél Zerquera Palacios, interview by López Blanch, *Historias Secretas*, 36–37.

35. Dr. Justo Piñeiro Fernández, interview by Don Fitz, February 9, 2016, Havana.

36. Dr. Domingo Díaz Delgado, interview by López Blanch, *Historias Secretas*, 132.

37. Gleijeses, *Conflicting Missions*, 213.

38. Dr. Diego Lagomasino Comesaña, interview by López Blanch, *Historias Secretas*, 59–60.

39. Dr. Héctor Vera Acosta, interview by López Blanch, *Historias Secretas*, 43.

40. Dr. Domingo Díaz Delgado, interview by López Blanch, *Historias Secretas*, 120.

41. Dr. Héctor Vera Acosta, interview by López Blanch, *Historias Secretas*, 42.

42. Dr. Amado Alfonso Delgado, interview by López Blanch, *Historias Secretas*, 144–46.

43. Dr. Rodrigo Álvarez Cambras, interview by López Blanch, *Historias Secretas*, 80.

44. Dr. Amado Alfonso Delgado, interview by López Blanch, *Historias Secretas*, 144.

45. Dr. Julián Álvarez Blanco, interview by López Blanch, *Historias Secretas*, 90.

46. Dr. Domingo Díaz Delgado, interview by López Blanch, *Historias Secretas*, 140.

47. Dr. Virgilio Camacho Duverger, interview by López Blanch, *Historias Secretas*, 158.

48. Dr. Rodrigo Álvarez Cambras, interview by López Blanch, *Historias Secretas*, 78.

49. Dr. Domingo Díaz Delgado, interview by López Blanch, *Historias Secretas*, 123.

50. Gleijeses, *Conflicting Missions*, 202.

51. Dr. Amado Alfonso Delgado, interview by López Blanch, *Historias Secretas*, 142.

52. Dr. Juan Antonio Sánchez, interview by Don Fitz, February 9, 2016, Havana, Cuba.

53. Dr. Héctor Vera Acosta, interview by López Blanch, *Historias Secretas*, 52.

54. Dr. Virgilio Camacho Duverger, interview by López Blanch, *Historias Secretas*, 161.

55. Dr. Amado Alfonso Delgado, interview by López Blanch, *Historias Secretas*, 142–48.

56. Ibid., 148.

57. Dr. Domingo Díaz Delgado, interview by López Blanch, *Historias Secretas*, 127.

58. Gleijeses, *Conflicting Missions*, 44, 201; Dr. Rafaél Zerquera Palacios, interview by López Blanch, *Historias Secretas*, 29.

59. Dr. Héctor Vera Acosta, interview by López Blanch, *Historias Secretas*, 48; Gleijeses, *Conflicting Missions*, 44, 168, 201.

60. Gleijeses, *Conflicting Missions*, 151.

61. Dr. Domingo Díaz Delgado, interview by López Blanch, *Historias Secretas*, 123; Dr. Julián Álvarez Blanco, interview by López Blanch, *Historias Secretas*, 90; Dr. Justo Piñeiro Fernández, interview by Don Fitz, February 9, 2016, Havana.

62. Dr. Amado Alfonso Delgado, interview by López Blanch, *Historias Secretas*, 149–50.

63. Dr. Domingo Díaz Delgado, interview by López Blanch, *Historias Secretas*, 131–32.

64. Dr. Virgilio Camacho Duverger, interview by López Blanch, *Historias Secretas*, 160.

65. Dr. Rodrigo Álvarez Cambras, interview by López Blanch, *Historias Secretas*, 78.

66. Dr. Rodolfo Puente Ferro, interview by López Blanch, *Historias Secretas*, 99, 102–3, 105; Gleijeses, *Conflicting Missions*, 168.

67. Gleijeses, *Conflicting Missions*, 169; Dr. Rodrigo Álvarez Cambras, interview by López Blanch, *Historias Secretas*, 84.

68. Dr. Rodrigo Álvarez Cambras, interview by López Blanch, *Historias Secretas*, 84; Dr. Justo Piñeiro Fernández, interview by Don Fitz, February 9, 2016, Havana.

69. Dr. Domingo Díaz Delgado, interview by López Blanch, *Historias Secretas*, 123.

70. Gleijeses, *Conflicting Missions*, 168; Dr. Rodolfo Puente Ferro, interview by López Blanch, *Historias Secretas*, 104–5.

71. Dr. Julián Álvarez Blanco, interview by López Blanch, *Historias Secretas*, 93.

72. Dr. Rafaél Zerquera Palacios, interview by López Blanch, *Historias Secretas*, 33–34; Dr. Amado Alfonso Delgado, interview by López Blanch, *Historias Secretas*, 150.

73. Dr. Virgilio Camacho Duverger, interview by López Blanch, *Historias Secretas*, 158.

74. Dr. Domingo Díaz Delgado, interview by López Blanch, *Historias Secretas*, 130–33.

75. Dr. Amado Alfonso Delgado, interview by López Blanch, *Historias Secretas*, 150.

76. Dr. Virgilio Camacho Duverger, interview by López Blanch, *Historias Secretas*, 162.

77. Gleijeses, *Conflicting Missions*, 216.

78. See chapter 2.

79. Gleijeses, *Conflicting Missions*, 203.

80. Ibid., 204.

81. Ibid.

4. From *Policlínicos Comunitarios* to Family Medicine

1. Dr. Julio López Benítez, interview by Don Fitz, January 5, 2017.

2. José R. Ruíz Hernández, *Cuba, Revolución Social y Salud Pública (1959–1984)* (Havana: Editorial Ciencias Médicas, 2008), 22.

3. Ibid., 74.

4. Margaret Gilpin, "Update—Cuba: On the Road to a Family Medicine Nation," *Journal of Public Health Policy* 12/1 (Spring 1991): 83-103, https://link.springer.com/article/10.2307%2F3342781; https://doi.org/10.2307/ 3342781.

5. Ibid.; Ross Danielson, *Cuban Medicine* (New Brunswick, NJ: Transaction Books, 1979), 198; José Díaz Novás and José A. Fernández Socarrás, "From Municipal Polyclinics to Family Doctor-and-Nurse Teams," *MEDICC Review*, 1–9, appeared in Spanish in *Revista Cubano de General Integral* 5/4 (1989): 556–64.

6. Danielson, *Cuban Medicine*, 197, 203.

7. Gilpin, "Update—Cuba," 80; Díaz and Fernández, "From Municipal Polyclinics to Family Doctor-and-Nurse Teams," 6; Ruíz, *Cuba, Revolución Social y Salud Pública*, 22.

8. Díaz and Fernández, "From Municipal Polyclinics to Family Doctor-and-Nurse Teams," 4; Danielson, *Cuban Medicine*, 201; Gilpin, "Update—Cuba," 89.

9. López, interview by Don Fitz.

10. Danielson, *Cuban Medicine*, 201–4.

11. López, interview by Don Fitz.

12. Danielson, *Cuban Medicine*, 201–4.

13. Ibid., 201, 205–7.

14. Díaz and Fernández, "From Municipal Polyclinics to Family Doctor-and-Nurse Teams," 6–9; Danielson, *Cuban Medicine*, 201–5.

15. Gilpin, "Update—Cuba," 89.

16. Linda M. Whiteford and Lawrence G. Branch, *Primary Health Care in Cuba: The Other Revolution* (Lanham, MD: Rowman & Littlefield, 2008), 37–38.

17. Ruíz, *Cuba, Revolución Social y Salud Pública*, 77; Whiteford and Branch, *Primary Health Care in Cuba*, 44.

18. Berta L. Castro Pacheco et al., *Cuban Experience in Child Health Care: 1959-2006* (Havana: Ministry of Public Health, 2010), 14, 17.

19. Whiteford and Branch, *Primary Health Care in Cuba*, 28.

20. Castro, *Cuban Experience in Child Health Care*, 42–43.

21. Gilpin, "Update—Cuba," 90–91.

22. Díaz and Fernández, "From Municipal Polyclinics to Family Doctor-and-Nurse Teams," 3–4; Whiteford and Branch, *Primary Health Care in Cuba*, 20–22.

23. Whiteford and Branch, *Primary Health Care in Cuba*, 22.

24. Díaz and Fernández, "From Municipal Polyclinics to Family Doctor-and-Nurse Teams," 5.

25. Dr. Justo Piñiero Fernández, interview by Don Fitz, January 5, 2017; López, interview by Don Fitz.

26. Díaz and Fernández, "From Municipal Polyclinics to Family Doctor-and-Nurse Teams," 5–9; Gilpin, "Update—Cuba," 90.

27. Díaz and Fernández, "From Municipal Polyclinics to Family Doctor-and-Nurse Teams," 5.

28. Danielson, *Cuban Medicine*, 201–5.

29. Whiteford and Branch, *Primary Health Care in Cuba*, 23; Gilpin, "Update—Cuba," 97.

30. Whiteford and Branch, *Primary Health Care in Cuba*, 23; Howard Waitzkin and Theron Britt, "Changing the Structure of Medical

Discourse: Implications of Cross-National Comparisons," *Journal of Health and Social Behavior* 30 (1989): 436–49; Howard Waitzkin et al., "Primary Care in Cuba: Low- and High-Technology Developments Pertinent to Family Medicine," *Journal of Family Practice* 45/3 (1997): 250–58; Gilpin, "Update—Cuba," 96.

31. Waitzkin, "Primary Care in Cuba," 252.

32. Gilpin, "Update—Cuba," 93, 98.

33. Ibid., 93–94.

34. Waitzkin and Britt, "Changing the Structure of Medical Discourse," 441; Gilpin, "Update—Cuba," 94; Ruíz, *Cuba, Revolución Social y Salud Pública,* 86.

35. Whiteford and Branch, *Primary Health Care in Cuba,* 28–29.

36. Danielson, *Cuban Medicine,* 205; John M. Kirk and Michael H. Erisman, *Cuban Medical Internationalism: Origins, Evolution and Goals* (New York: Palgrave Macmillan, 2009), 115.

37. Gilpin, "Update—Cuba," 94.

38. López, interview by Don Fitz.

39. Díaz and Fernández, "From Municipal Polyclinics to Family Doctor-and-Nurse Teams," 7.

40. Waitzkin and Britt, "Changing the Structure of Medical Discourse," 292.

41. Díaz and Fernández, "From Municipal Polyclinics to Family Doctor-and-Nurse Teams," 7.

42. Waitzkin, "Primary Care in Cuba," 250–54.

43. Candace Wolf, "The Zen of Healing: Two Surgeons Speak, Spoken Histories of Dr. José Gilberto Fleites Batista and Dr. Gilberto Fleites Gonzalez," unpublished ms., Havana, Cuba, January 2013.

44. Ruíz, *Cuba, Revolución Social y Salud Pública,* 88.

45. Wolf, "The Zen of Healing."

46. Waitzkin and Britt, "Changing the Structure of Medical Discourse," 423.

47. Ibid.

48. Whiteford and Branch, *Primary Health Care in Cuba,* 33.

49. Ibid.,

50. Gilpin, "Update—Cuba," 98.

51. Waitzkin and Britt, "Changing the Structure of Medical Discourse," 441.

52. Ibid., 442.

53. Navarro, "Health Planning in Cuba," 414.

54. Whiteford and Branch, *Primary Health Care in Cuba,* 24.

55. Gilpin, "Update—Cuba," 99.

56. Waitzkin and Britt, "Changing the Structure of Medical Discourse," 442.

57. Ibid., 445–47.

58. Ruíz, *Cuba, Revolución Social y Salud Pública*, 77; Whiteford and Branch, *Primary Health Care in Cuba*, 44.

59. Díaz and Fernández, "From Municipal Polyclinics to Family Doctor-and-Nurse Teams," 9.

60. López, interview by Don Fitz.

5. Cuban Doctors in Angola

1.   Piero Gleijeses, *Conflicting Missions: Havana, Washington, and Africa, 1959–1976* (Chapel Hill: University of North Carolina Press, 2002), 233. My account of Cuban participation in Angola relies heavily on the work of Piero Gliejeses, whose detailed, fascinating, and scholarly books comprise the definitive history of political and military campaigns in southern Africa during this period.

2.   Piero Gleijeses, *Visions of Freedom: Havana, Washington, Pretoria, and the Struggle for Southern Africa, 1976–1991* (Chapel Hill: University of North Carolina Press, 2013), 78.

3.   Gleijeses, *Conflicting Missions*, 381.

4.   See chapter 3.

5.   Gleijeses, *Conflicting Missions*, 245.

6.   Ibid., 251, 281, 285.

7.   Gleijeses, *Conflicting Missions*, 276; Gleijeses, *Visions of Freedom*, 28.

8.   Gleijeses, *Conflicting Missions*, 250.

9.   Ibid., 252, 266.

10. Ibid., 26, 276–77, 320, 341.

11. Ibid., 338, 340.

12. Gleijeses, *Visions of Freedom*, 34.

13. Gleijeses, *Conflicting Missions*, 376.

14. See chapter 1.

15. Gleijeses, *Visions of Freedom*, 15, 19.

16. Gleijeses, *Conflicting Missions*, 381.

17. Ibid., 380.

18. Hedelberto López Blanch, *Historias Secretas de Médicos Cubanos* (Havana: Centro Cultural de la Torriente Brau, 2005): Dr. Abigaíl Dambai Torres, interview by López Blanch, *Historias Secretas*, 201.

19. Ibid., 203.

20. Ibid., 205–7.

21. Ibid., 208–10.

22. Dr. Pedro Luis Pedroso Fernández, interview by López Blanch, *Historias Secretas*, 171–78.

23. Ibid., 179.

24. Ibid., 180.

25. Ibid., 181–82.
26. Ibid., 183.
27. Ibid., 184.
28. Ibid., 185.
29. Ibid., 178.
30. Dr. Omar Prudencio Martínez Herrera, interview by López Blanch, *Historias Secretas,*187–91.
31. Ibid., 187–89.
32. Ibid., 190.
33. Ibid., 191.
34. Ibid., 190.
35. Gleijeses, *Visions of Freedom*, 35, 39–56, 215.
36. Ibid., 60–62, 67, 157; Gleijeses, *Conflicting Missions,* 273.
37. Gleijeses, *Visions of Freedom*, 186–89, 221–26.
38. Gleijeses, *Conflicting Missions,* 270; Gleijeses; *Visions of Freedom*, 10, 66, 161, 248, 309–10.
39. Gleijeses, *Conflicting Missions,* 253; Gleijeses; *Visions of Freedom*, 300.
40. Gleijeses, *Visions of Freedom*, 301; Dr. Oscar Mena Hector, interview by Don Fitz, December 21, 2013, and January 1, 2014, Havana.
41. Gleijeses, *Visions of Freedom*, 302.
42. Ibid., 304.
43. Gleijeses, *Conflicting Missions,* 295; Gleijeses, *Visions of Freedom*, 209, 470.
44. Gleijeses, *Conflicting Missions,* 277; Gleijeses, *Visions of Freedom*, 178, 290–91.
45. Gleijeses, *Visions of Freedom*, 91, 326.
46. Ibid., 81–82, 84, 215, 333, 517–18.
47. Ibid., 81, 327.
48. Ibid., 78.
49. Mena, interview by Don Fitz.
50. Gleijeses, *Visions of Freedom*, 109; Mena, interview by Don Fitz.
51. Dr. Carlos Suárez Monteagudo, interview by Don Fitz, June 27, 2019, Havana.
52. Ibid.; Suárez, interview by Don Fitz.
53. Jorge Luís Martínez and Angel Chang, interview by Don Fitz, February 8, 2016, Havana.
54. Gleijeses, *Visions of Freedom*, 109, 329–33. The letters that Dr. Lourdes Franco Codinach wrote to her mother, and later provided to Gleijesis, are a remarkable portrait of Cuban aid workers' daily life in Angola. Dr. Franco believed that if the Cuban brigade head knew that they were shopping in the *candonga* nothing would have happened, despite rules having been broken. This shows why historians supplement

written rules and data with interviews whenever they can. Recounting of formal rules show how people are *supposed* to act while interviews suggest their *actual* behavior.

55. Gleijeses, *Visions of Freedom*, 328–32.

56. Ibid., 331–32.

57. Ibid., 329–31.

58. Ibid., 327–28.

59. Candace Wolf, "The Zen of Healing: Spoken Histories of Dr. José Gilberto Fleites Batista and Dr. Gilberto Fleites Gonzalez," unpublished manuscript sent to me by the author, January 2013, Havana, Cuba.

60. Gleijeses, *Visions of Freedom*, 29.

61. Ibid., 112, 191.

62. Ibid., 110, 191–92, 233–35.

63. Ibid., 339.

64. Ibid., 95, 262–63, 334, 385, 458, 477.

65. Ibid., 88, 331, 334; Mena, interview by Don Fitz.

66. Gleijeses, *Visions of Freedom*, 516; Gleijeses, *Conflicting Missions*, 228, 392; John M. Kirk and Michael H. Erisman, *Cuban Medical Internationalism: Origins, Evolution and Goals* (New York: Palgrave Macmillan, 2009), 68–69, 71.

67. Kirk and Erisman, *Cuban Medical Internationalism*, 74–75; Gleijeses, *Visions of Freedom*, 325.

68. Kirk reports that when "Ben Bella's government was overthrown in June 1965 . . . Havana's first foray into medical diplomacy came to an end." But Gliejeses writes, "The medical mission in Algeria continued without interruption" with a staff that fluctuated between thirty and sixty. Kirk and Erisman, *Cuban Medical Internationalism*, 68, 70; Gleijeses, *Conflicting Missions*, 228; Gleijeses, *Visions of Freedom*, 326–27.

69. Kirk and Erisman, *Cuban Medical Internationalism*, 76–77.

70. Ibid., 78–80.

71. Ibid., 68–69, 77, 79–81.

72. Gleijeses, *Visions of Freedom*, 326, 518.

73. Ibid., 68–69; Alexey V. Yablokov, Vassily B. Nesterenko, and Alexey V. Nesterenko, "Chernobyl: Consequences of the Catastrophe for People and the Environment," *Annals of the New York Academy of Sciences* 1181 (December 2009); John M. Kirk, *Health Care without Borders: Understanding Cuban Medical Internationalism* (Gainesville: University Press of Florida, 2015), 241–52; Kirk and Erisman, *Cuban Medical Internationalism*, 68–96; Gleijeses, *Visions of Freedom*; Dr. Julio López Benítez, *"Memorias de un Médico Cubano,* unpublished manuscript given to Don Fitz by the author, June 2013, Havana, 99.

74.   Ibid., 326, 392, 515; Kirk and Erisman, *Cuban Medical Internationalism*, 82.

75.   Gleijeses, *Visions of Freedom*, 356.

76.   Ibid., 367–99.

77.   Ibid., 397–99.

78.   Ibid., 405–11, 477.

79.   Ibid., 421–26.

80.   Ibid., 421, 426–27.

81.   Ibid., 462, 463, 466, 470–81.

82.   Ibid., 499–500.

83.   Ibid., 484–85.

84.   Ibid., 521; data for this table was obtained from the following web sites: https://www.populationpyramid.net/united-states-of-america/1975/, https://www.populationpyramid.net/cuba/1974/, and; http://www.answers.com/Q/How_many_US_military_served_during_Vietnam_War.

85.   Ibid., 494.

6. A Time of the Unexpected

1.   Tim Anderson, "HIV/AIDS in Cuba: A Rights-Based Analysis," *Health and Human Rights in Practice* 11/1 (2009): 93–104, https://cdn2.sph.harvard.edu/wp-content/uploads/sites/13/2013/07/10-Anderson.pdf, 96.

2.   Ibid., 97; Linda M. Whiteford and Lawrence G. Branch, *Primary Health Care in Cuba: The Other Revolution* (Lanham. MD: Rowman & Littlefield, 2008), 79; Nancy Scheper-Hughes, "AIDS, Public Policy, and Human Rights in Cuba," *The Lancet* 342/8877 (October 16, 1993): 965–67, https://doi.org/10.1016/0140-6736(93)92006-F.

3.   Whiteford and Branch, *Primary Health Care in Cuba*, 78.

4.   Anderson, "HIV/AIDS in Cuba: A Rights-Based Analysis," 96; Tim Anderson, "HIV/AIDS in Cuba: Lessons and Challenges," *Revista Panamericana de Salud Pública* 26/1 (2009): 78–86. doi: 10.1590/S1020-49892009000700012.

5.   Whiteford and Branch, *Primary Health Care in Cuba*, 78.

6.   Anderson, "HIV/AIDS in Cuba: A Rights-Based Analysis," 94.

7.   Ibid., 96.

8.   Ibid., 93–95; Anderson, "HIV/AIDS in Cuba: Lessons and Challenges," 81.

9.   Julia E. Sweig, *Cuba: What Everyone Needs to Know* (New York: Oxford University Press, 2009), 127–28; John M. Kirk and Michael H. Erisman, *Cuban Medical Internationalism: Origins, Evolution and Goals* (New York: Palgrave Macmillan, 2009), 98–99.

10.   John M. Kirk, *Health Care without Borders: Understanding Cuban*

Medical Internationalism (Gainesville: University Press of Florida, 2015), 240; Sweig, *Cuba*, 133–34; Kirk and Erisman, *Cuban Medical Internationalism*, 98–99, 122; Kamran Nayeri and Cándido M. López-Pardo, "Economic Crisis and Access to Care: Cuba's Health Care System Since the Collapse of the Soviet Union," *International Journal of Health Services* 35/4 (2005), 798–99. https://doi.org/10.2190/C1QG-6Y0X-CJJA-863H,

11. Nayeri and López-Pardo, "Economic Crisis and Access to Care," 798–99; Kirk and Erisman, *Cuban Medical Internationalism*, 46.

12. Nayeri and López-Pardo, "Economic Crisis and Access to Care," 798–99, 806; Kirk and Erisman, *Cuban Medical Internationalism*, 46, 99; Sweig, *Cuba*, 127–28, 143–44; Anderson, "HIV/AIDS in Cuba: Lessons and Challenges," 82.

13. Nayeri and López-Pardo, "Economic Crisis and Access to Care," 798–99, 807; Sweig, *Cuba*, 14344.

14. Dr. Julio López Benítez, interview by Don Fitz, June 28, 2019, Havana.

15. Nayeri and López-Pardo, "Economic Crisis and Access to Care," 798–99, 807; Piero Gleijeses, *Conflicting Missions: Havana, Washington, and Africa, 1959–1976* (Chapel Hill: University of North Carolina Press, 2002), 393.

16. Nayeri and López-Pardo, "Economic Crisis and Access to Care," 798.

17. Jane Franklin, *Cuba and the U.S. Empire: A Chronological History* (New York: Monthly Review Press, 2016), 364; Nayeri and López-Pardo, "Economic Crisis and Access to Care," 813.

18. Sweig, *Cuba*, 134; Kirk and Erisman, *Cuban Medical Internationalism*, 101.

19. Sweig, *Cuba*, 136; Kirk and Erisman, *Cuban Medical Internationalism*, 101.

20. Sweig, *Cuba*, 137.

21. Nayeri and López-Pardo, "Economic Crisis and Access to Care," 799.

22. Kirk and Erisman, *Cuban Medical Internationalism*, 101.

23. Ibid., 48, 102.

24. Ibid., 48–49.

25. Faith Morgan, Eugene "Pat" Murphy, and Megan Quinn, *The Power of Community: How Cuba Survived Peak Oil*, February 25, 2006. https://www.communitysolution.org/mediaandeducation/films/powerofcommunity

26. Whiteford and Branch, *Primary Health Care in Cuba*, 31.

27. Berta L. Castro Pacheco et al., *Cuban Experience in Child Health Care: 1959–2006* (Havana: Ministry of Public Health, 2010), 24–27.

28. Nayeri and López-Pardo, "Economic Crisis and Access to Care," 811; Kirk and Erisman, *Cuban Medical Internationalism*, 47.

29. Kirk and Erisman, *Cuban Medical Internationalism*, 47; Nayeri and López-Pardo, "Economic Crisis and Access to Care," 811–13; Kirk, *Health Care without Borders*, 147.

30. López Benítez, interview by Don Fitz.

31. Kirk, *Health Care without Borders*, 147; Kirk and Erisman, *Cuban Medical Internationalism*, 47; Nayeri and López-Pardo, "Economic Crisis and Access to Care," 803, 813; Castro Pacheco, *Cuban Experience in Child Health Care*, 24–25.

32. Sweig, *Cuba*, 146–47; Anderson, "HIV/AIDS in Cuba: A Rights-Based Analysis," 99. This encouragement has continued to be the case, as I noticed during my first trip to Cuba in 2009 when we chose a *consultorio* at random to enter and the first poster greeting us showed two men and gave the message to use condoms.

33. Whiteford and Branch, *Primary Health Care in Cuba*, 79; Sweig, *Cuba*, 146–47; Anderson, "HIV/AIDS in Cuba: Lessons and Challenges," 80, 82; López Benítez, interview by Don Fitz; Anderson, "HIV/AIDS in Cuba: A Rights-Based Analysis," 101.

34. Anderson, "HIV/AIDS in Cuba: A Rights-Based Analysis," 97; Anderson, "HIV/AIDS in Cuba: Lessons and Challenges," 83–84. The survey reports that, among the sixteen workers dismissed following HIV treatment, one discouraged worker gave up his appeal, but the other eleven with permanent jobs all kept them. Unfortunately, the four workers with temporary contracts lost their positions.

35. Candace Wolf, "The Zen of Healing: Spoken Histories of Dr. José Gilberto Fleites Batista and Dr. Gilberto Fleites Gonzalez," unpublished manuscript, January 2013, Havana, Cuba.

36. Ibid.

37. Scheper-Hughes, "AIDS, Public Policy, and Human Rights in Cuba"; Whiteford and Branch, *Primary Health Care in Cuba*, 79.

38. Anderson, "HIV/AIDS in Cuba: A Rights-Based Analysis," 98.

39. Whiteford and Branch, *Primary Health Care in Cuba*, 39, 77; Anderson, "HIV/AIDS in Cuba: Lessons and Challenges," 78–79.

40. Anderson, "HIV/AIDS in Cuba: A Rights-Based Analysis," 101; Anderson, "HIV/AIDS in Cuba: Lessons and Challenges," 83–84.

41. Anderson, "HIV/AIDS in Cuba: Lessons and Challenges," 85; Sweig, *Cuba*, 146–47; Whiteford and Branch, *Primary Health Care in Cuba*, 77; Chandler Burr, "Assessing Cuba's Approach to Contain AIDS and HIV," *The Lancet* 350/9078 (August 30, 1997): 647, doi:https://doi.org/10.1016/S0140-6736(05)63342-9.

42. Sweig, *Cuba*, 146-147; Kirk, *Health Care without Borders*, 301n6.

43. Anderson, "HIV/AIDS in Cuba: Lessons and Challenges," 83–84; Anderson, "HIV/AIDS in Cuba: A Rights-Based Analysis," 100.

44. Nayeri and López-Pardo, "Economic Crisis and Access to Care," 803–4; Castro Pacheco, *Cuban Experience in Child Health Care*, 24–25.

45. Nayeri and López-Pardo, "Economic Crisis and Access to Care," 803.

46. Date for Table 6.1 is from the following source: http://apps.who.int/gho/data/node.main.525?lang=en.

47. Whiteford and Branch, *Primary Health Care in Cuba*, 30, 56–57; Nayeri and López-Pardo, "Economic Crisis and Access to Care," 806.

48. López Benítez, interview by Don Fitz.

49. Nayeri and López-Pardo, "Economic Crisis and Access to Care," 805–6; Castro Pacheco, *Cuban Experience in Child Health Care*, 29; Whiteford and Branch, *Primary Health Care in Cuba*, 31.

50. Whiteford and Branch, *Primary Health Care in Cuba*, 75–76. While I am not a fan of spraying pesticides, I should note that those living in Havana during the spraying told me that it is done at periods corresponding to the lifecycle of mosquitoes in order to have the biggest effect, while timing of spraying in the United States seems to match political demands to "do something" rather than any biological understanding of the target species.

51. Nayeri and López-Pardo, "Economic Crisis and Access to Care," 809.

52. Date for Table 6.2 is from the following sources: https://www.worldlifeexpectancy.com/country-health-profile/cuba; https://www.worldlifeexpectancy.com/country-health-profile/united-states.

53. Kirk, *Health Care without Borders*, 236–52.

54. López Benítez, interview by Don Fitz.

55. Kirk, *Health Care without Borders*, 120; Kirk and Erisman, *Cuban Medical Internationalism*, 10–12; Gleijeses, *Conflicting Missions*, 393.

56. Kirk, *Health Care without Borders*, 119–38; Kirk and Erisman, *Cuban Medical Internationalism*, 129.

57. Kirk, *Health Care without Borders*, 119–38; Kirk and Erisman, *Cuban Medical Internationalism*, 129–31.

58. Kirk and Erisman, *Cuban Medical Internationalism*, 51–53, 128; Kirk, *Health Care without Borders*, 119–38.

59. Kirk and Erisman, *Cuban Medical Internationalism*, 53.

60. Kirk, *Health Care without Borders*, 124–38.

61. Sweig, *Cuba*, 145; Kirk, *Health Care without Borders*, 295n7.

7. ELAM: The Latin American School of Medicine

1. Steve Brouwer, "The Cuban Revolutionary Doctor: The Ultimate Weapon of Solidarity," *Monthly Review* 60/8 (January 2009): 28–42.

2. John M. Kirk and Michael H. Erisman, *Cuban Medical Internationalism: Origins, Evolution and Goals* (New York: Palgrave Macmillan, 2009), 128, 168.

3.   Escuela Latinoamericana de Medicina (ELAM), http://elacm.sld.cu/
     index.
4.   Exa Gonzales, interview by Don Fitz, December 28, 2009, in flight over
     the Gulf of Mexico.
5.   Brouwer, "The Cuban Revolutionary Doctor," 28–42.
6.   All information on Haiti is from Emily J. Kirk and John M. Kirk, "Cuban
     Medical Aid to Haiti: One of the World's Best Kept Secrets," *Synthesis/
     Regeneration: A Magazine of Green Social Thought* 53 (Fall 2010) 44–
     47.
7.   Ibid., 44–47.
8.   Ibid., 44–47.
9.   Escuela Latinoamericana de Medicina (ELAM), http://elacm.sld.cu/
     index.html.
10. Kirk and Erisman, *Cuban Medical Internationalism,* 3, 169, 112.
11. Ana Fernández Assán, Escuela Latinoamericana de Medicina (ELAM),
     http://elacm.sld.cu/index.html.
12. Ketia Brown, interview by Don Fitz, May 31, 2010, Havana.
     Information on YAB was also obtained from the document provided
     by Omavi Bailey: Yaa Asantewaa Brigade, August 15–September
     5, 2010. *African Medical Corps—Ghana Proposal,* Latin American
     School of Medicine, Carretera Panamericana 3 ½ KM, Santa Fe, Playa,
     Havana, CP 19142, Unpublished manuscript. For information on the
     Organization of African Doctors, see http://africanmedicalcorps.com.
     http://birthingprojectusa.org/.
13. Ibid., 2.
14. Cliff DuRand, "Humanitarianism and Solidarity Cuban-Style," *Z
     Magazine*, November 2007, 44–47.
15. Interview with Ketia Brown and document on Yaa Asantewaa Brigade,
     6.
16. Ibid.
17. Ibid., 7.
18. Linda M. Whiteford and Laurence G. Branch, *Primary Health Care in
     Cuba: The Other Revolution* (Lanham: Rowman & Littlefield, 2008), 2.
19. Emily J. Kirk and John M. Kirk, "Cuban Medical Aid to Haiti."
20. Brouwer, "The Cuban Revolutionary Doctor."
21. Interview with Nancy Remón Sánchez, ELAM, May 30, 2010.
22. Wuilmaris Pérez Torres, interview by Don Fitz, May 30, 2010, Havana.
23. Ivan Angulo Torres, interview by Don Fitz,, May 31, 2010, Havana.
24. On the role of the *consultorio* in the Cuban health system, see Lee
     T. Dresang, Laurie Brebick, Danielle Murray, Ann Shallue, and Lisa
     Sullivan-Vedder, "Family Medicine in Cuba: Community-Oriented
     Primary Care and Complementary and Alternative Medicine," *Journal*

of the American Board of Family Medicine 18/4 (July–August 2005): 297-303.

25. Dr. Alejandro Fadragas Fernández and Maité Perdomo, interview by Don Fitz, *Consultorio* No. 5, December 30, 2009, Havana.

26. Ketia Brown, interview by Don Fitz, May 31, 2010, Havana.

27. Cassandra Cusack Curbelo, interview by Don Fitz, January 23, 2010, Havana.

28. Anmnol Colindres, interview by Don Fitz, May 26, 2010, Havana.

29. Amanda Louis, interview by Don Fitz, May 28, 2010, Havana.

30. Dennis Pratt, interview by Don Fitz, May 26, 2010, Havana.

31. Jonalisa Livi Tapumanaia, interview by Don Fitz, May 28, 2010, Havana.

32. Lorine Auma, interview by Don Fitz, June 2, 2010, Havana.

33. Keitumetse Joyce Letsiela, interview by Don Fitz, June 2, 2010, Havana.

34. Dresang et al., "Family Medicine in Cuba."

35. Ivan Gomez de Assis, interview by Don Fitz, May 27, 2010, Havana.

36. Walter Titz, interview by Don Fitz, June 2, 2010, Havana.

37. Interview with Yell Eric, ELAM, June 2, 2010.

38. For detailed information on ELAM, current curriculum for U.S. students, and an application, see https://ifconews.org/cuba-caravan/.

39. Rebecca Fitz and Ivan Angulo Torres, interview by Don Fitz, June 3, 2010, Havana.

8. Thirteen Faces of ELAM

1. For information on the "brain drain," see John M. Kirk and H. Michael Erisman, *Cuban Medical Internationalism: Origins, Evolution and Goals* (New York: Palgrave Macmillan, 2009); and Margaret G. Zackowitz, "Village Health Workers," *National Geographic* (December 2008): 156.

2. In 2010 there were 3,406 pre-med, first-year, and second-year students living at the main ELAM campus near Havana and 6,169 third-year through sixth-year students in the Havana area, for a total of 9,675 students attending the school. The total had climbed to over 11,000 students from 123 countries in 2014. [John M. Kirk, *Health Care without Borders: Understanding Cuban Medical Internationalism* (Gainesville, FL: University Press of Florida, 2015), 43] During the two decades of its existence, ELAM has graduated over 30,000 doctors. This figure is from http://www.cubadebate/cu/noticias/2019/09/03/elam-ejemplo-de-so.

9. Cuba: The New Global Medicine

1. John M. Kirk and Michael H. Erisman, *Cuban Medical Internationalism* (New York: Palgrave Macmillan, 2009).

2. Ibid., 112, 120, 169.

3.   Steve Brouwer, *Revolutionary Doctors* (New York: Monthly Review Press, 2011).

4.   Rebecca Fitz, interview by Don Fitz, St. Louis, Missouri, August 1, 2011.

5.   Lucien Chauvin, "Recovering from the Peru Earthquake," *Time*, August 20, 2007.

6.   Núcleo del PSR en Cuba, Nuestra Misión (Nucleus of the Peruvian Socialist Revolutionary Party in Cuba), *Nuestra Misión* (unreleased video), 2007.

7.   Leopoldo García Mejias, interview by Don Fitz, Pisco, Peru, December 27, 2010.

8.   One *sol* equals about 36 cents.

9.   Dr. Johnny Carrillo Prada and Dr. María Concepción Paredes Huacoto, interview by Don Fitz, Pisco, Peru, December 27, 2010.

10. Leticia Martínez Hernández, "Joanna, una rebelde con causa," *Digital Granma Internacional*, April 12, 2010, http://granma.cubaweb.cu.

11. See Project Bonafide, "Vision," http://projectbonafide.com.

12. Originally designated at the "Henry Reeve International Team of Medical Specialists in Disasters & Epidemics," they have come to be known as the "Henry Reeve Brigades." Joanna Souers, phone interviews by Don Fitz, February 21, 2011, and July 9, 2011. For more on the Henry Reeve Brigade, see Conner Gory, "Cuban Disaster Doctors in Guatemala, Pakistan," *MEDICC Review* 7/9 (November–December 2005): 11–12.

13. Bill Quigley, "Haiti Facts Seventeen Months After Earthquake," *ZNet*, June 26, 2011, http://zcommunications.org.

14. Emily J. Kirk and John M. Kirk, "Cuban Medical Aid to Haiti: One of the World's Best Kept Secrets," *Synthesis/Regeneration* 53 (Fall 2010), 44-47.

15. The Sri Lanka tsunami of December 26, 2004, resulted in 40,000 deaths and 2.5 million people being displaced. See "Worst Ever Tragedy in Sri Lanka History," http://lankalibraray.com.

16. An example of Cuba's dealing with gross medical negligence is the 2011 trial in which the prosecutor asked for six- to fourteen-year sentences for doctors, nurses, and other professionals accused of causing respiratory illnesses and deaths of psychiatric patients by inadequately protecting them from unusually cold weather conditions in January 2010. See José A. de la Osa, "Havana Psychiatric Hospital Trial Concludes," *Digital Granma Internacional*, January 24, 2011, http://granma.cu.

17. Yaa Asantewaa Brigade, "African Medical Corps—Ghana Proposal," August 15–September 5, 2010 (unpublished report).

18. "Yaa Asantewaa," *Born Black Magazine* 3 (February 2009), http://bornblackmag.com.

19.   Much of what they saw is available on YouTube in three short films: *Healing: African Medical Corps*: Part 1, Part 2 and Part 3, www.youtube. com.

20.   Omavi Bailey, "Yaa Asantewaa Medical Brigade," December 2010 (unpublished report).

21.   Omavi Bailey, interviews by Don Fitz, July 15 and 29, 2011.

22.   See chapter 7.

23.   Bailey, "Yaa Asantewaa Medical Brigade."

24.   For effects of the U.S. embargo see Amnesty International U.S.A., *The US Embargo Against Cuba: Its Impact on Economic and Social Rights*, September 2, 2009, http://amnestyusa.org.

25.   Linda M. Whiteford and Laurence G. Branch, *Primary Health Care in Cuba* (Lanham, MD: Rowman & Littlefield, 2008), 31.

10. Challenges of the Twenty-First Century

1.   Steve Brouwer, *Revolutionary Doctors: How Venezuela and Cuba Are Changing the World's Conception of Health Care* (New York: Monthly Review Press, 2011), 69.

2.   Ibid., 63–65.

3.   Ibid., 89.

4.   Ibid.

5.   Ibid., 131.

6.   Ibid., 87.

7.   Ibid., 91.

8.   Ibid., 97.

9.   Ibid., 84.

10.   Ibid., 140.

11.   The fifteen-member group who participated in MEDICC's "Gender and Health Care" program that year included a MEDICC coordinator from the United States and a translator, liaison, and medical consultant from Cuba.

12.   Cuban health professionals use *"pesquizaje activa"* to mean "active screening" when they go door-to-door. Conner Gorry, email to author, January 24, 2012.

13.   Paulo Lázaro et al., "Assessment of Human Health Vulnerability to Climate Variability and Change in Cuba," *MEDICC Review* 10/2 (Spring 2008): 1–9.

14.   "Dengue fever, A.D.A.M.," *Medical Encyclopedia, PubMed Health*, http://www.ncbi.nlm.nih.gov/pubmedhealth/PMH0002350/.

15.   "Dengue hemorrhagic fever, A.D.A.M." *Medical Encyclopedia, PubMed Health*, http://www.ncbi.nlm.nih.gov/pubmedhealth/PMH0002349/ http://www.ncbi.nlm.nih.gov/pubmedhealth/PMH0002349/.

16. Dengue fever entry, *Medical Encyclopedia, PubMed Health*.

17. Dengue hemorrhagic fever entry, *Medical Encyclopedia, PubMed Health*, http://www.ncbi.nlm.nih.gov/pubmedhealth/PMH0002349/.

18. V. Vanlerberghe et al., "Community Involvement in Dengue Vector Control: Cluster Randomized Trial," *MEDICC Review* 12/1 (Winter 2010): 41–47, https://www.medigraphic.com/pdfs/medicreview/mrw-2010/mrw101i.pdf.

19. Vanlerberghe, "Community Involvement in Dengue Vector Control"; Lázaro, "Assessment of Human Health Vulnerability," 41.

20. Linda Whiteford and Lawrence G. Branch, *Primary Health Care in Cuba: The Other Revolution*. (Lanham, MD: Rowman & Littlefield, 2008); Lázaro, "Assessment of Human Health Vulnerability," 5.

21. See chapter 7.

22. Whiteford and Branch, *Primary Health Care in Cuba, 25*.

23. "Medical Education Cooperation with Cuba," http://www.medicc.org/ns/index.php?s=3&p=3; Maria G. Guzmán and Gustavo Kouri, "Dengue Haemorrhagic Fever Integral Hypothesis: Confirming Observations, 1987–2007," *Transactions of the Royal Society of Tropical Medicine and Hygiene* 102/6 (July 2008): 522–23, DOI: 10.1016/j.trstmh.2008.03.001.

24. Otto Peláez et al., "Prevalence of Febrile Syndromes in Dengue Surveillance, Havana City, 2007," *MEDICC Review* 13/2 (April 2011): 47–51, https://www.researchgate.net/publication/51202690_Prevalence_of_febrile_syndromes_in_dengue_surveillance_Havana_City_2007; Cristina Díaz et al., "Estrategía Intersectoral y Participativa con Enfoque de Ecosalud para la Prevención de la Transmisión de Dengue en el Nivel Local," *Cadernos Saúde Pública* 25, Supl. 1 (2009): S59S70, http://dx.doi.org/10.1590/S0102-311x2009001300006; V. Vanlerberghe, "Community Involvement in Dengue Vector Control,"41–42.

25. V. Vanlerberghe, "Community Involvement in Dengue Vector Control," 45.

26. Don Fitz, "Eight Reasons U.S. Healthcare Costs 96% More Than Cuba's—With the Same Results," December 9, 2010, http://www.alternet.org/health/149090/eight_reasons_us_healthcare_costs_96%25_more_than_cuba%27s--with_the_same_results.

27. L. T. Dresang et al., "Family Medicine in Cuba: Community-Oriented Primary Care and Complementary and Alternative Medicine," *Journal of the American Board of Family Medicine* 18/4 (July–August 2005): 297–303. DOI:https://doi.org/10.3122/jabfm.18.4.297.

28. Richard S. Cooper et al., "Health in Cuba," *International Journal of Epidemiology* 35/4 (August 1, 2006): 817–24, https://doi.org/10.1093/ije/dyl175.

29. J. Pérez, "Gender and HIV Prevention," slide presentation at the Pedro Kouri Institute of Topical Medicine, Havana, May 15, 2012.

30. Linda Whiteford and Lawrence G. Branch, *Primary Health Care in Cuba: The Other Revolution* (Lanham, MD: Rowman & Littlefield, 2008), 79.

31. John M. Kirk and Michael H. Erisman, *Cuban Medical Internationalism: Origins, Evolution and Goals* (New York: Palgrave Macmillan, 2009), 188.

32. See chapter 7.

33. Kirk and Erisman, *Cuban Medical Internationalism*, 13–14, 25, 117, 129.

34. Cooper, "Health in Cuba."

11. Cuba's Medical Mission

1. John M. Kirk, *Health Care without Borders: Understanding Cuban Medical Internationalism* (Gainesville, FL: University Press of Florida, 2015), 58.

2. Ibid., 118.

12. Medicine in Cuba and the United States

1. Conner Gorry, "Cuba's Family Doctor-and-Nurse Teams: A Day in the Life," *MEDICC Review*, 19, no. 1 (January 2017), 6-9.

2. See chapter 7.

3. Gorry, "Cuba's Family Doctor-and-Nurse Teams," 6.

4. Ibid.

5. Don Fitz, lecture at Washington University in St. Louis, April 14, 2011.

6. Ibid.

7. Gorry, "Cuba's Family Doctor-and-Nurse Teams," 7.

8. Fitz, lecture at Washington University.

9. Gorry, "Cuba's Family Doctor-and-Nurse Teams," 6.

10. Fitz, lecture at Washington University.

11. Gorry, "Cuba's Family Doctor-and-Nurse Teams," 9.

12. Berta L. Castro Pacheco et al., *Cuban Experience in Child Health Care: 1959–2006* (Havana: Ministry of Public Health, 2010). 39.

13. Gorry, "Cuba's Family Doctor-and-Nurse Teams," 8–9.

14. Steffie Woolhandler, David U. Himmelstein, and Adam Gaffney, "Single Payer Is Actually a Huge Bargain," *The Nation*, August 10, 2018, https://www.thenation.com/article/single-payer-actually-huge-bargain/.

15. Robert Pollin et al., *Economic Analysis of Medicare for All* (Political Economy Research Institute: University of Massachusetts Amherst, November 30, 2018), https://www.peri.umass.edu/component/k2/item/1127-economic-analysis-of-medicare-for-all

16. Dean Baker, "Medicare for All Act: Testimony Before House Rules Committee," *CounterPunch*, May 3, 2019, https://www.counterpunch.org/2019/05/03/medicare-for-all-act-testimony-before-house-rules-committee/

17. Melissa Hellmann, "U.S. Health Care Ranked Worst in the Developed World," *Time*, June 17, 2014, time.com/2888403/u-s-health-care-ranked-worst-in-the-developed-world/?utm_source=emailshare&utm_medium=email&utm_campaign=email-share-article&utm_content=20190429.

18. Pete Dolack, "The Cost of Not Having Single Payer: $1.4 Trillion Per Year," *CounterPunch*, July 14, 2017, https://www.counterpunch.org/2017/07/14/the-cost-of-not-having-single-payer-1-4-trillion-per-year/.

19. Associated Press, "A look at medical costs in Cuba vs. the U.S.," *Modern Healthcare*, August 27, 2012, https://www.modernhealthcare.com/article/20120827/INFO/308279923/a-look-at-medical-costs-in-cuba-vs-the-u-s.

20. L. T. Dresang et al., "Family Medicine in Cuba: Community-Oriented Primary Care and Complementary and Alternative Medicine," *Journal of the American Board of Family Medicine,* 18, no 4 (July–August, 2005) 297–303.

21. John M. Kirk and Michael H. Erisman, *Cuban Medical Internationalism: Origins, Evolution and Goals* (New York: Palgrave Macmillan, 2009), 182.

22. "Which healthcare system would you rather work in: Cuba or USA?, " Brighton School of Business and Management, June 19, 2018, https://www.brightonsbm.com/news/healthcare-systems-compared/.

23. J. A. Harrison, "Paying More, Getting Less: How Much Is the Sick US Health Care System Costing You?" *Dollars & Sense,* May/June, 2008, http://dollarsandsense.org/archives/2008/0508harrison.html

24. S. Woolhandler et al., "Cost of Health Care Administration in the United State and Canada," *New England Journal of Medicine*, 349, no. 8 (August 21, 2003): 768–775.

25. Baker, "Medicare for All Act."

26. Woolhandler, Himmelstein, and Gaffney, "Single Payer Is Actually a Huge Bargain."

27. Baker, "Medicare for All Act."

28. Dean Baker, "Health Care Costs and the Budget," *CounterPunch*, March 7, 2019, https://www.counterpunch.org/2019/03/07/health-care-costs-and-the-budget/.

29. Edward M. Murphy, "The Real Driver of Health Care Spending," *CommonWealth*, July, 9, 2018, https://commonwealthmagazine.org/opinion/the-real-driver-of-health-care-spending/#.

30. Ralph Nader, "25 Ways the Canadian Health Care System is Better than Obamacare," December 28, 2018, https://www.counterpunch. org/2018/12/28/25-ways-the-canadian-health-care-system-is-better-than-obamacare/.

31. P. J. Devereaux et al., "Payments for Care at Private For-Profit and Private Not-for-Profit Hospitals: A Systematic Review and Meta-analysis," *Canadian Medical Association Journal*, 170, no. 12 (June 8, 2004), 1817–24. DOI: 10.1503/cmaj.1040722.

32. A. P. Wilper et al., "Hypertension, Diabetes, and Elevated Cholesterol among Insured and Uninsured U.S. adults," *Health Affairs,* w1151–w1159.

33. R. D. Quint, *You Bet Your Life: Why We Need a National Health Program,* Slide show presented in Havana, Cuba (May 2010). Emergency Room costs can be complicated by the expenses a hospital incurs when it has difficulty finding an empty bed for moving a new patient into.

34. Nicholas Kristof, "Why Infants May Be More Likely to Die in America Than Cuba," *The New York Times*, Section SR (January 19, 2019), 11. https://www.nytimes.com/2019/01/18/opinion/sunday/cuba-health care-medicare.html.

35. Stan Cox, *Sick Planet: Corporate Food and Medicine* (Ann Arbor: Pluto Press, 2008), 1.

36. Ibid.

37. Ibid.

38. Ibid.

39. Martha Rosenberg, "Pharma 'Screening' Is a Ploy to Seize More Patients," *CounterPunch*, July 20, 2018, https://www.counterpunch. org/2018/07/20/pharma-screening-is-a-ploy-to-seize-more-patients/

40. Martha Rosenberg, *Born with a Junk Food Deficiency: How Flaks, Quacks, and Hacks Pimp the Public Health* (Amherst, NY: Prometheus Books, 2012), 148.

41. Rosenberg, "Pharma 'Screening.'"

42. Rosenberg, *Born with a Junk Food Deficiency,* 43-47.

43. B. E. Levine, "Review of Robert Whitaker's *Anatomy of an Epidemic,*" *Z Magazine*, 23, no. 9 (September 2010) 36–37.

44. Rosenberg, *Born with a Junk Food Deficiency,* 70.

45. Claudia Wallis, "Why Fake Operations Are a Good Thing," *Scientific American,* 318, no. 2, (February 2018): 22, https://www. scientificamerican.com/article/how-fake-surgery-exposes-useless-treatments/ doi:10.1038/scientificamerican0218-22.

46. Karin Meissner et al., "Differential Effectiveness of Placebo Treatments: A Systematic Review of Migraine Prophylaxis," *Journal of the American Medical Association Intern Med.*, 173, no. 21 (November 25, 2013): 1941–

1951, https://www.ncbi.nlm.nih.gov/pubmed/24126676 doi:10.1001/jamainternmed.2013.10391.

47. Claudia Wallis, "Why Fake Operations Are a Good Thing."

48. Rachelle Buchbinder et al., "A Randomized Trial of Vertebroplasty for Painful Osteoporotic Vertebral Fractures," *New England Journal of Medicine*, 361, (August 6, 2009): 557–568, https://www.nejm.org/doi/full/10.1056/NEJMoa0900429#t=article DOI: 10.1056/NEJMoa0900429.

49. Rasha Al-Lamee et al., "Percutaneous Coronary Intervention in Stable Angina (ORBITA): A Double-blind, Randomised Controlled Trial," *The Lancet*, 391, no. 10115 (January 6, 2018) 31–40, DOI:https://doi.org/10.1016/S0140-6736(17)32714-9.

50. Claudia Wallis, "Why Fake Operations Are a Good Thing."

51. J. LaForge, "Oversight of Dangerous High-dose Medical Radiation," *Z Magazine*, 23 no. 7/8 (July/August 2010): 10–11.

52. M. W. Moyer, "Heartburn Headache," *Scientific American*, 303, no. 1 (July 2010): 24–26.

53. Rosenberg, *Born with a Junk Food Deficiency*, 52.

54. Ibid., 73.

55. Ibid.

56. Ibid., 43–44.

57. Ibid., 73, 80.

58. Cox, *Sick Planet*.

59. Ralph Nader. "Gross Hospital Negligence Does Not Exempt Celebrities," *In the Public Interest*, September 26, 2018, https://nader.org/2018/09/26/gross-hospital-negligence-does-not-exempt-celebrities/.

60. Kate Yoder, "If U.S. Health Care Were a Country, It Would Rank 13th for Emissions," *Grist*, June 14, 2016, https://grist.org/climate-energy/if-u-s-health-care-were-a-country-it-would-rank-13th-for-emissions/?utm_medium=email&utm_source=newsletter&utm_campaign=daily-horizon.

61. Matthew J. Eckelman and Jodi Sherman, "Environmental Impacts of the U.S. Health Care System and Effects on Public Health," *PLOS ONE*, June 9, 2016, 1–14 https://journals.plos.org/plosone/article?id=10.1371/journal.pone.0157014 https://doi.org/10.1371/journal.pone.0157014.

62. Ziba Kashef, "Environmental and Health Impacts of U.S. Healthcare System," *YaleNews*, June 9, 2016, https://news.yale.edu/2016/06/09/environmental-and-health-impacts-us-healthcare-system.

63. Yoder, "If U.S. Health Care Were a Country, It Would Rank 13th for Emissions."

64. *Injury Facts*, vistited July 12, 2019, https://injuryfacts.nsc.org/motor-vehicle/overview/introduction/.

65. Rosenberg, *Born with a Junk Food Deficiency*, 204.

66. Ibid., 207.

67. Martha Rosenberg, "Proof That the Pharma Business Model Actually Wants People Sick," *AlterNet*, March 6, 2017; https://www.alternet.org/2017/03/pharma-funded-patient-groups-keep-drug-prices-astronomical/.

68. Rosenberg, *Born with a Junk Food Deficiency*, 152–154.

69. B. Abrahamsen et al., "Patient Level Pooled Analysis of 68,500 Patients from Seven Major Vitamin D Fracture Trials in US and Europe," *British Medical Journal*, 340 (January 12, 2010): b5463, https://www.ncbi.nlm.nih.gov/pmc/articles/PMC2806633/ doi: 10.1136/bmj.b5463.

70. Rosenberg, *Born with a Junk Food Deficiency*, 152–154.

71. Ibid., 26–27.

72. Ibid., 31.

73. Irving Kirsch et al., "Initial Severity and Antidepressant Benefits: A Meta-Analysis of Data Submitted to the Food and Drug Administration," *PLOS Medicine*, 5, no. 2 (February 26, 2008): e45. https://journals.plos.org/plosmedicine/article?id=10.1371/journal.pmed.0050045 doi:10.1371/journal.pmed.0050045.

74. Leonard Sax, *Boys Adrift: The Five Factors Driving the Growing Epidemic of Unmotivated Boys and Underachieving Young Men* (New York: Basic Books, 2007).

75. Gary Stix, "Turbocharging the Brain." *Scientific American*, 301 no. 4 (October 2009): 46–49, 52–55.

76. Rosenberg, *Born with a Junk Food Deficiency*, 51.

77. Ibid., 64.

78. Joseph Stiglitz, "A Rigged Economy," *Scientific American,* 319, no 5 (November, 2018): 56–61, https://www.scientificamerican.com/article/the-american-economy-is-rigged/?redirect=1 doi:10.1038/scientificamerican1118-56.

79. Fran Quigley, "Corporations Killed Medicine. Here's How to Take It Back," *TheNation.com*, February 12, 2016, https://www.thenation.com/article/corporations-killed-medicine-heres-how-to-take-it-back/.

80. Baker, "Medicare for All Act."

81. Murphy, "The Real Driver of Health Care Spending."

82. Baker, "Medicare for All Act."

83. Baker, "Health Care Costs and the Budget."

84. Dean Baker, "Is Globalization to Blame?" *Boston Review*, January 9, 2017, https://bostonreview.net/forum/dean-baker-globalization-blame.

85. Marshall Allen, "The Myth of Drug Expiration Dates," *ProPublica*, July 18, 2017, https://www.propublica.org/article/the-myth-of-drug-expiration-dates .

86. Ibid.

87. Lyon et al., "Stability Profiles of Drug Products Extended beyond Labeled Expiration Dates," *Journal of Pharmaceutical Sciences,* 95, no. 7 (July 2006): 1549–1560, https://www.documentcloud.org/documents/3525372-Stability-Profiles-of-Expired-Drugs.html   DOI 10.1002/jps.20636.

88. Lee Cantrell et al., "Stability of Active Ingredients in Long-Expired Prescription Medications," *Archives of Internal Medicine,* 172, no. 21, (November 26, 2012): 1685–687, https://www.documentcloud.org/documents/3516397-Expired-drugs-research-letter.html doi:10.1001 / archinternmed.2012.4501

89. Allen, "The Myth of Drug Expiration Dates."

90. Ibid.

91. José R. Ruíz Hernández, *Cuba, Revolución Social y Salud Pública (1959–1984)* (*Editorial Ciencias Médicas*: La Habana, Cuba, 2008), 15–16, 63; Ross Danielson, *Cuban Medicine.* (New Brunswick: Transaction Books, 1979), 158, 171.

92. Baker, "Health Care Costs and the Budget."

93. Ibid.

94. Baker, "Is Globalization to Blame?"

95. Ibid. Baker claims that negative effects of bringing doctors from poor countries could "be offset by taxing the income of foreign professionals and repatriating it to their home countries, which could use that money to train two or three professionals for every one lost to the United States." This is a convoluted Ponzi scheme that fails to acknowledge that the two or three doctors being trained in poor countries would themselves want to come to the United States, thereby increasing the damage with each round of doctor-attraction.

96. Emma Court and Lydia Ramsey, "Healthcare CEOs Make as Much as $26 Million a Year. Here's What the Industry's Top Executives Earned in 2018." *Business Insider,* May 16, 2019, https://www.businessinsider.com/pharma-and-healthcare-ceo-compensation-2018-2019-4.

97. Court and Ramsey, "Healthcare CEOs Make as Much as $26 Million a Year."

98. Christine Willmsen and Martha Bebinger, "Lawsuit Details How the Sackler Family Allegedly Built an OxyContin Fortune," *National Public Radio, Inc.,* February 1, 2019, https://www.npr.org/sections/health-shots/2019/02/01/690556552/lawsuit-details-how-the-sackler-family-allegedly-built-an-oxycontin-fortune.

99. S. Woolhandler, D. U. Himmelstein, and M. Amberg, *Over 2,200 Veterans Died in 2008 Due to Lack of Health Insurance,* Physicians for a National Health Program Press Release (November 10, 2009).

100. P. J. Devereaux et al., "A Systematic Review and Meta-analysis of Studies Comparing Mortality Rates of Private For-profit and Private Not-for-profit Hospitals," *Canadian Medical Association Journal*, 166, no. 11, (May 28, 2002): 1399–1406, http://www.cmaj.ca/content/166/11/1399.

101. David U. Himmelstein et al., "Quality of Care in Investor-owned vs. Not-for-profit HMOs," *Journal of the American Medical Association*, 282, no. 2 (July 14, 1999): 159–163, http://www.pnhp.org/sites/default/files/docs/Quality-of-Care-at-Investor-Owned-Himmelstein.pdf doi:10.1001/jama.282.2.159.

102. Nader, "25 Ways the Canadian Health Care System Is Better than Obamacare."

103. Ibid.

104. Pierre Chirac and Els Torreele, "Global Framework on Essential Health R&D," *The Lancet*, 367, no. 9522 (May 13, 2006): 1560–1561, https://www.thelancet.com/journals/lancet/article/PIIS0140-6736(06)68672-8/fulltext DOI:https://doi.org/10.1016/S0140-6736(06)68672-8.

105. Fran Quigley, "Corporations Killed Medicine."

106. Kathryn Hall-Trujillo, interview by Don Fitz, September 21, 2018.

107. Birthing Project USA: Model Programs, https://www.birthingproject usa.org/model-programs.html Visited July 13, 2019.

108. Kathryn Hall-Trujillo, interview by Don Fitz.

109. Sarpoma Sefa-Boakye M.D., interview by Don Fitz, October 4, 2018.

110. Sarpoma Sefa-Boakye M.D., interview by Don Fitz.

Postscript: How Che Guevara Taught Cuba To Confront Covid-19

1. See https://www.cuartopoder.es/internacional/2020/03/21/cuba-tiem pos-coronavirus-pascual-serrano/.

2. See https://www.counterpunch.org/2020/04/10/cuban-medical-science -in-the-service-of-humanity/.

3. See https://www.counterpunch.org/2020/04/09/john-lennon-in-quarantine-a-letter-from-havana/.

4. See https://boletinaldia.sld.cu/aldia/2020/04/12/medicamento-homeo patico-a-ciudadanos-en-cuba/.

5. See https://www.resumen-english.org/2020/04/door-by-door-the-cub an-government-delivers-immune-boosting-medicine-to-the-people/

6. See https://venezuelanalysis.com/analysis/14834.

7. See https://www.telesurenglish.net/news/Venezuela-Has-the-Lowest-Contagion-Rate-in-Latin-America-20200414-0012.html.

8. See https://www.mintpressnews.com/ecuador-unable-to-cope-with-coronavirus-imf-measures/266570/.

9. See https://www.nytimes.com/aponline/2020/04/03/world/europe/ap-cb-virus-outbreak-cuban-doctors.html .

10. See http://en.granma.cu/cuba/2020-04-16/the-covid-19-pandemic-makes-clear-the-need-to-cooperate-despite-political-differences.

11. See https://www.resumen-english.org/2020/04/cuba-interferon-saves-lives/.

12. See https://countercurrents.org/2020/04/undaunted-cuba-defies-the-empire-and-extends-hands-of-solidarity-to-continents.

13. See https://www.thenation.com/article/world/coronavirus-cuba-cruise-ship/.

14. See https://www.democracynow.org/2020/3/24/cuba_medical_diplomacy_italy_coronavirus.

15. See https://www.thenation.com/article/world/coronavirus-cuba-cruise-ship/.

16. See http://links.org.au/cuba-contribution-to-combating-covid-19.

17. See https://www.telesurenglish.net/news/more-than-40-nations-ask-cuba-for-interferon-alpha-b-20200327-0004.html.

18. See https://indypendent.org/2020/04/cuban-trained-doctor-helps-mobilize-pandemic-response-in-her-south-bronx-community/.

INDEX

192; *consultorios* and, 89, 220–
23; doctor-nurse teams in, 77,
81, 83, 205; doctors in, 77, 79,
83; family medicine and, 82–83,
89; from *policlínicos integrales*
to, 75–80; teamwork in, 77–78;
vaccination campaigns of, 79
policlínicos integrales, 39–42,
52–53, 89; CDRs and, 47; centralization, decentralization
and, 43–45; decentralization
and, 46–48; doctors on, 42, 45,
48, 75–76; health campaigns
coordinated by, 46; hospitals
and, 44–45; MINSAP and, 40,
44–45, 76; mobilization and,
45–48; to *policlínico comunitario*, 75–80; problems with,
75–76, 79–80; specialists in,
75–76
polio, 36, 40, 68–70, 72–73, 202–3
Polymerase Chain Reaction
(PCR), 250, 253
polypharmacy, 230
Popular Armed Forces for the
Liberation of Angola (FAPLA),
93–94, 96, 103, 113, 119–21
Popular Movement for the
Liberation of Angola (MPLA),
91–94, 119–20, 122
Portugal, 91–93
Powell, Colin, 132
The Power of Community, 134
Pratt, Dennis, 160–61, 173
Préval, René, 153
PrevengHo-Vir, 249
preventive medicine, 27, 40, 48,
83, 108, 199–200; MGI and,
195, 205; U.S. and, 227

primary care, 41, 89, 136, 145
Primary Health Care in Cuba
(Whiteford and Branch), 191
private practices, of Cuban doc-
tors, 42–43
profit-based medicine, 238–40
Programa Integral de Salud
(Comprehensive Health
Program), 152
Prolia (firm), 234
ProPublica, 237
proton pump inhibitors (PPIs),
230
Puente, Rodolfo, 60, 69
Purdue Pharma (firm), 238

Quibala (Angola), 98, 100
Quigley, Fran, 235

race: in African conflicts, 58; of
Cuban military doctors and
troops, in Africa, 58–60;
medical revolution and,
35–36
racism, 35; anti-racist struggle
against, 95, 113–14; in medicine, 87; Savimbi's pact with,
103–5; of white regimes in
Africa, 58, 114
radiation, 229–30
Reagan, Ronald, 91, 102–5, 117,
120–21
Red Cross, 46
Reformista, of FMC, 24
Renovación, of FMC, 24
Resik Habib, Pablo, 32–33
Resno Albara, José, 34
Revolutionary Doctors (Brouwer),
180